The
Healing Power
of Resilience

The Healing Power *of* Resilience

A NEW PRESCRIPTION FOR HEALTH AND WELL-BEING

TARA NARULA, MD

Simon Element
*New York   Amsterdam/Antwerp   London
Toronto   Sydney/Melbourne   New Delhi*

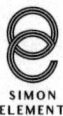
SIMON
ELEMENT

An Imprint of Simon & Schuster, LLC
1230 Avenue of the Americas
New York, NY 10020

For more than 100 years, Simon & Schuster has championed authors and the stories they create. By respecting the copyright of an author's intellectual property, you enable Simon & Schuster and the author to continue publishing exceptional books for years to come. We thank you for supporting the author's copyright by purchasing an authorized edition of this book.

No amount of this book may be reproduced or stored in any format, nor may it be uploaded to any website, database, language-learning model, or other repository, retrieval, or artificial intelligence system without express permission. All rights reserved. Inquiries may be directed to Simon & Schuster, 1230 Avenue of the Americas, New York, NY 10020 or permissions@simonandschuster.com.

Copyright © 2026 by Tara Narula Cangello

All rights reserved, including the right to reproduce this book or portions thereof in any form whatsoever. For information, address Simon Element Subsidiary Rights Department, 1230 Avenue of the Americas, New York, NY 10020.

First Simon Element hardcover edition January 2026

SIMON ELEMENT is a trademark of Simon & Schuster, LLC

Simon & Schuster strongly believes in freedom of expression and stands against censorship in all its forms. For more information, visit BooksBelong.com.

For information about special discounts for bulk purchases, please contact Simon & Schuster Special Sales at 1-866-506-1949 or business@simonandschuster.com.

The Simon & Schuster Speakers Bureau can bring authors to your live event. For more information or to book an event, contact the Simon & Schuster Speakers Bureau at 1-866-248-3049 or visit our website at www.simonspeakers.com.

Interior design by Silverglass

Manufactured in the United States of America

10 9 8 7 6 5 4 3 2 1

Library of Congress Control Number: 2025945817

ISBN 978-1-9821-9884-8
ISBN 978-1-6682-2546-2 (Int Exp)
ISBN 978-1-9821-9885-5 (ebook)

To Siena and Layla: my greatest blessings.
My love is with you forever.
Shine your bright lights, seek the silver linings,
stay resilient, and savor every single day.

To Dave: my lobster.
I love you with all my heart.
It's you and me together, always.

To my parents: my roots.
Always grateful for and love you both.
You taught me to dream, have faith, and
believe anything is possible.

It matters not how strait the gate,
how charged with punishments the scroll,
I am the master of my fate,
I am the captain of my soul.

—William Ernest Henley

Contents

Introduction xi

CHAPTER 1
The Origins of the Resilience Response 1

CHAPTER 2
Why Stress Is the Heart of the Matter 17

CHAPTER 3
Accept Your Current Situation 41

CHAPTER 4
Embrace Flexible Thinking 63

CHAPTER 5
Get Fit 87

CHAPTER 6
Face Your Fear 117

Contents

CHAPTER 7

Build Connections 139

CHAPTER 8

Seek Out Love 167

CHAPTER 9

Finding Hope and Having Faith 191

CHAPTER 10

Pursue Your Purpose 211

Epilogue 235

Acknowledgments 237

Notes 241

Index 255

Introduction

The human heart is a wondrous organ. It is the biological engine that keeps us alive, pumping blood throughout our bodies, without cessation, until we take our last breath. Its design is intricate, its component parts fragile, and yet, it's a miracle of reliable engineering.[1] We can hear its rhythmic work and we can feel it beating in our chest. But most of us forget that it's even there.

What so captivates me about this fist-size organ, weighing barely ten ounces and working, literally, around the clock, is this: Why does it work so flawlessly for so long for some, and yet fail, often without warning, for others? And how is it that it is able to continue functioning well, even after being seriously diseased or damaged, allowing a person to continue to live a full, rich, and meaningful life?

The mysteries of the human heart are what led me in my residency to specialize in cardiology. I wanted to understand what could cause a heart to falter or fail and then—either through medical intervention, or a lifestyle change, or a combination of both—be restored to full functionality. I wanted to know how this organ could be replaced,

Introduction

wholesale, by the donation of the organ by another and then carry on and sustain an entirely new and different life.

I am now a noninvasive cardiologist; I see patients of all ages with cardiovascular issues ranging from the potentially concerning to the life-threatening. I consciously chose to leave the inpatient setting several years ago so that I can follow my patients further on their journey. When I see individual patients year after year, I get to know them as people and can offer a continuity of care that isn't possible when you are treating people only in the operating room or the hospital.

I am also a medical journalist; I am fascinated by people's stories, and in seeing how sharing them can help all of us "get better," whether by learning something new about health or inspiring us to make a change. I often report about stories of the heart and many other medical topics.

In both my medical practice and my reporting I have wondered, again and again, What makes the human heart so resilient?

The human heart weighs between eight and ten ounces. It beats, on average, about one hundred thousand times a day or about seventy-five times a minute (that's safely more than two billion times over an eighty-year lifespan). It has its own electrical system, which prompts it to pump, on average, about two thousand gallons of blood a day. This requires a lot of energy and oxygen, as each pump of the heart exerts pressure roughly equivalent to squeezing a tennis ball. This pressure causes the heart to contract, sending blood coursing through a network of sixty thousand miles of blood vessels in the body, delivering oxygen and nutrients to all the body's cells, then returning to the heart via a network of veins. Here are a few other interesting facts about the heart that explain why I and so many others find it so fascinating:

Introduction

- A human aorta is about an inch in diameter, or roughly the size of a garden hose.
- The sound of the beating heart is the sound of its valves opening and closing.
- The first open-heart surgery was performed in the United States in 1893 by a Black cardiologist named Daniel Hale Williams.
- The heart will continue to beat—even when it is removed from the body—as long as it has an oxygen supply.
- A broken heart is a real phenomenon and can mimic a heart attack. Fortunately, "broken heart" syndrome is rarely fatal.

And here's one more fact about the heart that explains why I've devoted my life to understanding it:

- In the United States, a person dies every thirty-four seconds from cardiovascular disease; with the most recent statistics, that translates into 941,652 people in a single year.

Cardiovascular disease kills more people than all forms of cancer and accidents combined. And new data indicates that by 2035, fully 45 percent of the US population will experience a heart-disease-related issue.

Modern medicine allows us to use imaging to combat heart disease, to detect blockages and assess congenital defects. We can make major adjustments to the heart's component parts by repairing its valves, performing bypass surgery, or implanting devices that will augment its ability to run smoothly. We've certainly made impressive advances in cardiovascular care, and yet . . .

Introduction

Despite these advances and our culture's obsession with health and wellness, we haven't been able to get heart disease under any sort of meaningful control, even though the rate of death by heart diseases has fallen some over the past seventy-five years. This frustrates me, and it should concern you, too. Clearly, we are not giving our hearts what they need to stay healthy and high functioning. Although we know with certainty some of the major causes of heart disease, other, less quantifiable factors are at play, and these are the factors that interest me the most. We know that a poor, processed-food-focused diet, smoking, and a lack of physical activity are contributors—but what else is at play? Only by getting a more comprehensive understanding of why our modern lifestyles are harming our hearts will we be able to heal.

My father is also a cardiologist. He is still practicing, even in his late eighties. He was one of the founders of cardiac electrophysiology, the field focused on understanding the electrical system of the heart. When I was in medical school, I decided early on that, although I wanted to follow in my father's footsteps and specialize in cardiology, I did not want to become a researcher, as he had; I also knew I did not want to be a surgeon. Sure, the mechanical aspects of the heart are fascinating to me, but what most interested me was building relationships with my patients, and taking care of their heart health more holistically. Rather than spend my days in a lab or in an operating room, I could have real relationships with patients I saw year after year through office visits, not just during procedures. As I mentioned, that's exactly what I do.

I truly want to know what makes my patients tick. The heart is a wondrous organ, but I don't *just* look at their hearts. I look at whole people, and understanding them as a whole is key to my work and to their medical outcomes. That's how I can look beyond those usual lifestyle factors. I ask them questions about their lives, and I listen to their answers. I want to

Introduction

understand what they are grappling with, so that I can then educate them and empower them to take control over their heart health.

I realized over the years in talking with my patients that their receiving a medical diagnosis or dealing with a change in their medical status was akin to—or sometimes represented—a traumatic event. Treating their medical condition was only one part of my directive as their doctor. I also wanted to help people learn how to navigate a medical challenge or trauma and deal with what was to come next—to help them move toward an appreciation and acceptance of the overall quality of the life they would have in its aftermath.

I've had patients come to me who had so little heart function that it was a miracle that they were able to walk into my office at all. But these patients were often the ones to make the most profound changes. Why was this so? I've also worked with patients who, with just a minor lifestyle adjustment, could have gotten their blood pressure under control, and yet sometimes these patients just aren't able to make what seems like a slight change. Again—why was this so? Why is it that some of my patients are able to rise to their health challenges in such an amazing way? And why are some, despite the presence of serious cardiac health issues, able to live a great life? These are the patients who fascinate me the most; I decided to explore what separates these patients and allows them to thrive in the face of adversity.

So I began to gather and examine my patients' stories, searching for some kind of common denominator that put them on a path of healing, even when overcoming an illness or managing a disease was no longer an option. What separates these patients is something that moves beyond the realm of physical health and moves into the territory of mental health. This is when I had that "Aha!" moment and realized that these patients were exhibiting a psychological strength

Introduction

that was influencing how they responded to a diagnosis or a treatment plan or even the end of life. I was beginning to understand that, just as the human heart is designed to be resilient and to withstand a fair amount of stress, so, too, is the human mind and spirit.

I started to take note of the ways in which my patients responded to a diagnosis or treatment plan. I also started to ask patients what they needed and desired in the face of a medical challenge. What they needed, it became clear, was a plan for building and strengthening resilience. In my office, my patients often wondered, "When will I feel like myself again?" And that helped me see how building and strengthening resilience might help them navigate the uncertainty of a diagnosis or treatment plan. What I began to observe intrigued me so much that I became a passionate student of resilience and the psychology of resilience. I wanted to understand how resilience might influence medical outcomes for my patients.

As I've mentioned, for many years, doctors have seen how lifestyle changes could affect cardiac health. Now, I was beginning to suspect that perhaps it was this aspect of their lifestyle—their psychological lifestyle, if you will—that might be the key ingredient. I knew there was something important here, that it needed to be examined and discussed, but it wasn't something that was easily quantifiable or easy to study in the ways that traditional medicine relies on. My work as a medical journalist pointed to that, too. Profiling so many individuals who have overcome trauma fascinated me. I realized there was a bridge that needed to be built between psychology research, resilience training, and clinical medical practice. These worlds need to be combined and connected, so I've set out to do it.

I'm going to talk about this word *resilience* a lot. For clarity's sake, I'd like to share my definition now. It is informed by my medical practice,

Introduction

my extensive research and medical journalism, and my fascination with how we overcome hardship, in health situations or otherwise.

First, a bit about what resilience is not. Resilience is not the capacity to return to the same place you began after trauma or tragedy. Neither our minds nor our bodies are built like rubber bands: We do not "bounce back." We are influenced and affected; we recover; we grow; we change. This, I believe, is what the core of resilience is: the ability to embrace change. Michelangelo is purported to have said, "I saw the angel in the marble and I carved until I set him free." We are constantly being shaped by our experiences, change affecting the composition as a whole even as we remain ourselves. We are the marble, and we are the angel.

I believe that resilience is what allows us to enjoy the daily experience of being alive, before, during, or in the aftermath of trauma or tragedy. As the tried-and-true saying goes, the only constant is change. Life is all about adapting to it. And if at a baseline you are unable to enjoy the daily experience of being alive, there's no bigger problem. Of course, when encountering trauma or tragedy it takes time to recover, and a new baseline may be required afterward. But it can be found—which is where resilience comes in. My objective with my patients is to help them build resilience, so that they embrace change and can enjoy the daily experience of being alive.

To dig deeper, I have found that to build resilience requires developing certain skills:

- an acceptance of your current situation
- a flexible mindset that can allow for change—especially important given that change is inevitable
- a commitment to pursuing physical health through lifestyle choices such as diet, exercise, and adequate rest

Introduction

- an ability to face fears
- a commitment to connecting with those who surround you in daily or more lasting ways
- embracing a love of self and others
- an optimistic or hopeful outlook on the future
- a feeling of or pursuit of purpose

With these ingredients, anyone can build resilience. This is what I call the Resilience Response.

As I already described, my first and primary focus as a doctor is on quality of life. I am not a psychologist, but I am a physician and a medical journalist, and I've spent the last decade recording my patients' stories in an effort to capture the connection between resilience and a positive medical outcome, even when the diagnosis is hard or even dire. I also became interested in understanding if building resilience might protect one's heart health and help forestall the onset of heart and other diseases. I began to see that resilience was not only essential to meeting the traumas, tragedies, challenges, and failures that we all must face, but it's essential to retaining one's sense of wonder, joy, and excitement about life. It is a critical tool to help in prevention of disease, too—so really, resilience is fostering prevention and treatment all in one.

Along with sharing the incredible stories of my own patients who have built resilience, I've interviewed experts who study resilience and who are adding to a growing body of research that will, I hope, begin to influence our understanding of how our physical health, mental health, and our spiritual fortitude are profoundly intertwined; because when we're talking about the body, mind, and spirit, we're actually talking about one thing, and one thing only: a living, breathing human being. And it is my hope that, one day, in the not-too-distant

Introduction

future, we physicians will truly understand how essential resilience is to healing for us living, breathing human beings. Resilience training should and can become part of the standard of care for patients and what we teach in medical school.

With that in mind, I've designed the heart of the book to include a comprehensive set of tools to educate and inspire and help you explore and build and rely on your own resilience.

More than anything else, I want you to come away from this book feeling motivated and empowered to cultivate resilience in your life in order to strengthen your heart, improve your health, and live the fullest life possible.

CHAPTER 1

The Origins of the Resilience Response

I was a sixteen-year-old intern in the University of Miami's cardiology department when I watched my first heart transplant. Draped in a baggy blue paper gown, I huddled up with several other interns at the back of Operating Room #2 as the patient was wheeled in. We had been told that her name was Anne, that she was forty-seven years old, married, and the mother of four. A massive heart attack had damaged her heart beyond repair. Without a transplant she would, we all understood, surely die.

I watched as the surgeon and his team opened the woman's chest and extracted what we knew was a dying organ. Then, with a steady, swift hand, he took the waiting donor heart and gently placed it into Anne's chest cavity. The next several hours would be spent painstakingly and meticulously attaching the new heart to her veins and arteries, but within minutes of the transplant, after being connected to the major blood vessels, it was beating steadily, and distributing blood throughout her body—nothing short of a miracle to witness. With this procedure, Anne had, quite literally, been given a new lease on life.

The Healing Power of Resilience

This was just the first of many times I have stood in awe at the power of the human body, specifically the human heart, to withstand great trauma, and yet . . . somehow survive.

What I glimpsed that day was resilience. When I think back on Anne and her transplant surgery, I can't help but think about what she faced. I'm sure she was advised that, without the transplant, she'd have no chance of living long enough to see her children grow up. I'm also certain that she was told that the transplant itself might fail, so she knew that the surgery was not without great risk.

Anne was faced with the kind of monumental decision that most of us, we hope, will never have to face. Yet . . . she had the resilience to go ahead with the surgery. She then not only survived it, but continues to thrive.

I have never forgotten what it felt like to see that insulated Styrofoam box arrive in the surgical room, knowing it contained the ultimate gift from another person, a gift of life. I have never forgotten what it felt like to see, for the first time, a human body made so vulnerable as during transplant surgery. Over the intervening years, I've thought a lot about Anne—not only her time on the operating table. I've also thought about some of the hurdles she had to overcome to prepare herself for such a high-stakes medical procedure—and recovery from it, as well.

I have found that to cultivate resilience requires developing certain skills, and with Anne I saw them on full display, one by one. First, acceptance of your current situation. Anne had to accept the truth of her medical condition. Absorbing the news that her heart was so damaged that it could no longer keep her alive must have been devastating, shocking; her proximity to her death became undeniable. This meant that she had to embrace that she was at a life-or-death moment. Next, a flexible mindset that can allow for change. Once Anne had accepted her current situation and her two options

The Origins of the Resilience Response

(do nothing and die or undergo a transplant and improve her odds of survival, but with no guarantees), she then made a choice: to undergo a transplant that would give her a chance to live and spend more time with her husband and kids, but would require an arduous surgery and a long recovery. Having a sense of purpose is a key ingredient in resilience, and certainly Anne's family helped her feel that in her life. Resilience also requires finding or maintaining an optimistic or hopeful outlook; choosing surgery meant that Anne would be putting her life into the hands of a team of highly skilled medical professionals, a group of people who were all but strangers to her. This meant she had to muster an incredible amount of hope and trust that these strangers could and would do everything they could to save her life. She also had to have hope that she could survive a difficult, risky surgery. Resilience also means a commitment to pursuing physical health through lifestyle choices such as diet, exercise, and adequate rest. I'm sure she was also prepped to understand that having open-heart surgery was extremely hard on the body, the mind, and the spirit, so she had, despite her rapidly deteriorating health, to muster a tremendous amount of strength and to plan ahead for a long, difficult recovery. Her family was ready to love and support her, adding to her ability to tackle the challenge. Anne would also have had to manage or put aside her fear, calling upon tremendous courage. Anne brought all these qualities into Operating Room #2 that day. And that was just the beginning.

Surviving massive heart surgery and recovering from a cardiac episode requires incredible resilience. But with the ingredients described above—acceptance, a flexible mindset, commitment to pursuing physical health, an ability to face fears, a feeling of or pursuit of purpose, and an optimistic or hopeful outlook, bolstered by the love and support of connections and community, whenever possible—anyone can cultivate resilience, no matter how big or small the challenge. This is what I call the Resilience Response.

Resilience, in Mind and Body and Spirit

As I mentioned in the introduction to this book, after any kind of medical trauma, one of the first questions a patient inevitably asks me is "When will I feel like myself again?"

To answer it I rely on my being a doctor first and a cardiologist second. After all, after a cardiac event people want assurances not only about heart health, but also about their health in general—physical, mental, spiritual. And as a doctor, I am concerned with the overall well-being of the person in front of me. My goal is to treat the person, not the body. And that means focusing on far more than the status of a single organ, no matter how essential that organ is to survival.

In my twenty-plus years as a doctor, I have noticed that something is missing in patient care: addressing mental health when we talk about physical health. The two are inextricably linked. I cannot tell you how many times I have entered an exam room to talk about heart failure or coronary artery disease and ended up talking about someone's state of mind before we get to their symptoms of shortness of breath or chest pain, or how I instinctually take note of the levels of hope and despair in someone's voice as much as their blood pressure or heart rate.

Believing you're able to meet the challenge of something as traumatic as massive heart surgery—trauma akin to that of a physical assault, a natural disaster, or a terrorist attack—is as essential to survival as any number measured by science. Our ability to respond and recover from trauma has mental components, along with physical ones. Medical interventions

The Origins of the Resilience Response

and even serious diagnoses, too, are forms of trauma—which is not readily recognized—and for many patients a healthcare event can haunt or psychologically paralyze them. This is just one way that the connection between mind and body is not being appropriately addressed.

So when people ask, "When will I feel like myself again?," I answer them candidly, and I talk about their whole selves, not just their hearts. I tell them, you may not feel like your same self again. You may well feel differently, perhaps permanently—like a new version of yourself, and that's not necessarily bad. You are starting a new chapter in a life that will be meaningful and happy, and perhaps even healthier than before. Again, it may be necessary to set a new baseline, with new expectations about what life will be like going forward. As we emerge from the challenges of life like the angel from the marble, we may look a bit different from what we previously imagined.

As I think back to Anne's experience, she had to release a failing organ and embrace a new one that was not her own. I cannot think of a more profound example of the miraculous resilience of the human body than this. Our bodies are truly wondrous compilations of organs that all work in concert and give us life.

Anne's body was resilient, and so was her mind and her spirit.

The mind is essential to supporting—and enhancing—the body's resilience. I've come to believe, based on my experience, the experiences of my patients, and my many conversations with experts in the field of resilience, that these two types of resilience—one physical, the other psychological—are intertwined. When we cultivate both—our body's resilience and our mind's and spirit's resilience—we position ourselves both to prevent the onset of illness or disease, and to restore our health when faced with either.

Based on my work as a doctor, a journalist, and a medical professional who has read widely in psychology and about health outcomes, I can confidently say that while there is a growing body of research on resilience, no one is putting all these elements together. Here I do so in a way that will equip patients and readers with the tools to build both types of resilience.

Psychological resilience is not a fixed trait that we're born with, such as the color of our eyes. It's a set of skills that every one of us has the capacity to develop throughout our lives. It's what allows us to meet challenges, from staying calm when we're being insulted or demeaned to, like Anne, preparing for massive heart surgery. Life is predictably unpredictable; every one of us will face failure, loss, and uncertainty in our lives, every one of us will suffer in ways big and small. But how we meet these events matters.

Physical resilience is our body's ability to overcome injury or disease. Factors such as age, genetics, and underlying medical conditions can hamper or support our body's ability to recover from accidents or illness. But physical resilience, too, is not fixed. It can be improved or degraded based on our lifestyle (exercise preferences, sleep habits, eating choices)—and it is also deeply connected to our mindset: Whether we have hope or despair about the future, for instance, will affect how we meet the events I describe above. There is evidence that a positive mindset can enhance immune responses, suggesting that optimism can buffer the body from the harmful effects of stress, which can impact physical health and recovery. A study on teenagers who regularly exercised found a connection between physical activity and psychological resilience. Exercising regularly can improve mental well-being for all of us, and for these teenagers, it also decreased their social sensitivity, which can in turn enhance resilience and the ability to cope with challenges. This connection, between psychological and physical resilience, is one we will explore in depth in this book.

The Origins of the Resilience Response

After practicing medicine for two decades and exploring these topics through my experiences with patients, through researching and writing, and through speaking with groups from the American College of Cardiology and the American Heart Association to the viewers of the morning news, I am more convinced than ever about the importance of and connection between psychological and physical resilience. While thankfully there is a growing body of research, there are still several missing pieces to put in place to solve the puzzle of how the two fit together. I am on the front lines of exciting developments that will help to complete that puzzle.

A Short History of Resilience Psychology

Before delving into those developments, we need to look back a bit on what scientific literature says about psychological resilience to date. The wisdom of acknowledging the connection between mind and body has been with us for a long time. Ancient philosophers such as the Stoics openly discussed it: The phrase *mens sana in corpore sano*, "a healthy mind in a healthy body," has held the test of time! But only quite recently, in the middle of the last century, has a more humanistic and holistic approach to patient care emerged in modern medicine. Around this time, clinicians became interested in the interplay among a patient's mental, emotional, and physical life, and an approach to wellness that addressed the impact of the body, mind, and spirit.

In the 1950s, psychologist and researcher Abraham Maslow coined the phrase *positive psychology* to describe the shift in psychology away from a focus on the "disordered"—in other words, seeing the person as something that needs to be "fixed"—to a new approach, which was interested in understanding how humans flourish. He advocated for observing how a patient expressed (or struggled to express) her potential, and then worked with a patient to first identify her natural coping abilities, then build on them, to achieve that potential.

Unlike the generations of psychologists before him, Maslow and other proponents of a more humanistic approach to psychology believed humans are hardwired for self-actualization. The old way of thinking often assumed a patient's coping abilities were set; this new way emphasized that a patient could improve them and therefore adapt well to the world around her. How she thought could change how she lived.

At roughly the same time, a young psychologist at Duke University named Norman Garmezy, who was focused on improving the quality of life of those diagnosed with schizophrenia, was the first to use the word *resilience* formally. His definition came from his groundbreaking research on how stress affects a child's competence and development. As he put it, resilience is "not necessarily impervious[ness] to stress. Rather, resilience is designed to reflect the capacity for recovery and maintained adaptive behavior that may follow initial retreat or incapacity upon initiating a stressful event." He made a career studying the resilience of children exposed to early child abuse, poverty, and schizophrenic parents. He created a theoretical framework for this—in other words, what combination of factors leads to resilience—that is still being applied to resilience research today. Take, for example, a 2020 study that found that children who grow up in harsh environments are able to develop skills that help them with adaptability—suggesting that adversity can actually lead to greater resilience. This is referred to as adaptive calibration or stress adaptation, the shaping of cognitive and behavioral development to promote survival in unpredictable or dangerous settings. It has its drawbacks, too, though. For example, these children learn to constantly scan their surroundings for potential threats, and thus they can develop

The Origins of the Resilience Response

a remarkable ability to detect subtle cues of danger. And this might lead to hypervigilance in situations where it is not warranted, taxing their stress response (more on this later). In other words, these skills honed in harsh environments may not be beneficial in every situation.

In another fascinating study across the Atlantic a child psychiatrist named Michael Rutter famously studied Romanian orphans who often spent extended periods with little social interaction or physical affection. Rutter (who collaborated with Garmezy on other occasions) showed a correlation between the duration of a child's stay in an orphanage and how well they faired once adopted. He compared Romanian children who came to the United Kingdom for adoption before the age of six months, and those who were adopted after, and found that the former were cognitively caught up to their UK-born peers by four, while the latter were not. By doing this, he demonstrated, empirically, that resilience is not a set psychological trait. If that were the case, a child would either be resilient or not—no matter the length of their stay in an orphanage: They would either show deleterious effects from the experience, or not. Though some of Garmezy's research focused on a particular population, he also found that childhood circumstances were not the sole contributor to the ability to be resilient. Rutter observed the same. He, like Garmezy, identified three key factors contributing to building resilience: the individual, the family, and the community. In other words, both Rutter and Garmezy identified one's individual personality, the quality of the immediate family structure, and the level of support from one's community as external factors that contribute to resilience, thereby dispelling the myth that resilience is a fixed personality trait.

Another early pioneer of resilience theory was Emmy Werner, a developmental psychologist who, along with Ruth Smith, launched a groundbreaking study on risk and resilience. They began studying all the babies (698) born on the Hawaiian island of Kauai in 1955. They followed this population for forty years and tracked their exposure to elements that would challenge their resilience (including everything from premature birth, to poverty, to being in a household under the care of a mentally ill parent, etc.). One of their findings showed that one-third of the highest-risk children exhibited resilience and were able to overcome the elements above and grow into self-confident, compassionate, and highly productive adults. The researchers also identified some of the factors that influenced resilience, such as having a mentor, a spiritual or religious community, hobbies, or physical activities. Werner, based on her studies of children, defined resilience as one's ability to "work well, play well, love well, and expect well."

As the field of resilience psychology has continued to blossom, and our understanding of how resilience can be strengthened has grown, the definition of resilience has taken on even more nuance. The late Steven Southwick, MD, a world-renowned expert on resilience and trauma, once defined resilience as "the ability to bend but not break, bounce back, and perhaps even grow in the face of adverse life experiences." He went on to say, "The more we learn about resilience, the more potential there is for integrating salient concepts of resilience into relevant fields of medicine, mental health, and science."

In the mid-1990s, two psychologists, Richard Tedeschi, PhD, and Lawrence Calhoun, PhD, posited a new theory, based on their research, that those who endure and persevere through trauma and adversity often experience not just personal growth, but *positive* personal growth. But this often comes with much struggle, hardship, and overcoming: "People develop new understandings of themselves, the world they live in, how to relate to other people, the kind of future they might have, and a better understanding of how to live life," Tedeschi has said.

The Origins of the Resilience Response

Tedeschi and Calhoun went on to create the Posttraumatic Growth Inventory (PTGI) to quantify the growth of trauma survivors.

More recently, I'm especially intrigued by the work of George Bonanno and Robert Galatzer-Levy, who was once a student of Bonanno's. Both have looked deeply at why some people are, or become, more resilient than others. Bonanno, a clinical psychologist at Columbia University, went in search of what factor or factors set these people apart. His theory of resilience, which he began constructing in the early 2000s, is built on the belief that we all share the same basic stress-response system, which helps us respond to stressors (more on that in the next chapter). But some of us are better at using this system. Why? Bonanno pinpointed *perception* as the key variable: people who frame adversity as an opportunity to grow can move through a stressful experience before it can become a traumatic one. This was a stunning breakthrough in understanding resilience. Bonanno learned that those who ground themselves, confident that they have the tools to handle a stressful experience, can prevent an experience from becoming harmful. (He called these stressful experiences PTEs, or potentially traumatic events.) His discovery highlighted an important aspect of resilience: the belief in one's ability to cope.

Starting in the 2010s, Galatzer-Levy, a professor of psychiatry and behavioral neuroscience at New York University, conducted various studies with Bonanno. The factors that bolster an individual's resilience, they found, are optimism and regulatory flexibility. Their focus was on people who suffered heart attacks, lung disease, heart disease, stroke, and cancer, as well as those who divorced, and they found that being depressed *before* the onset of the stressor did not correlate with a lack of resilience or an increased mortality rate, but becoming depressed *after* the stressful event did. In essence, we all possess the ability to be resilient, but some of us are better equipped to put this ability to use. Why would that be the case? Based on what he's learned so far, Bonanno does not believe that there is a genetic component to resilience, though he is finding that there is a genetic link to the kinds of psychopathology (depression, anxiety, PTSD, etc.) that may inhibit the expression of resilience.

Picking up on the work of Tedeschi and Calhoun and others, Dennis Charney, MD, a psychiatrist and neurobiologist who led the Mood and Anxiety Research Program at the National Institute of Mental Health, studied the effects of trauma on Navy SEALs, victims of sexual and physical abuse, and 9/11 first responders. His research among diverse populations cut across all ethnic, racial, and socioeconomic groups. From this work he developed a "prescription" for developing resilience.

Charney called his findings the 10 Essential Principles of Resilience. These include (1) being optimistic (but realistically so); (2) being cognitively flexible; (3) having a personal moral compass; (4) finding a role model; (5) facing fear; (6) actively using coping skills; (7) having a social support network; (8) exercising; (9) developing emotional intelligence; and (10) recognizing your strengths. Though Charney and I share some commonalities in how we conceive of resilience and what we recommend people do to develop and enhance it, we vary in our perspectives and advice. In the same way that doctors develop unique protocols for patients, with no two "prescriptions" exactly alike, his book comes from a psychologist's expertise while I use my background in cardiology to focus on people's health journeys, drawing on my clinical experience advising and treating patients, and also my time as a medical journalist.

And unfortunately, Charney had to put all of his resilience research into practical use when he himself faced a life-threatening trauma.

On one early August morning in 2017, Charney stopped at Lange's Little Store & Delicatessen in Chappaqua, New York, for his usual—an

The Origins of the Resilience Response

iced coffee and a bagel. It was just another day for Charney, who was headed in to his job as dean of the Icahn School of Medicine at Mount Sinai in Manhattan. Charney paid, grabbed his order, and stepped out of the store and onto the sidewalk. Almost immediately, he heard the blast of a shotgun, then looked down to see blood pouring from his shoulder. He turned and ran back into the store, screaming, "I've been shot!" He was, he later learned, the target of an assassination attempt by a disgruntled former employee who had been terminated, several years earlier, for falsifying research data. Charney did not know this man, but Charney's signature was on the termination letter.

Charney was rushed to Westchester Medical Center, where it was discovered that fifteen pellets had penetrated his shoulder, lung cavity, diaphragm, and the area around his liver. He lost half of his blood volume and was in the ICU for five days. As soon as he regained consciousness, he thought, "Okay. Time to find out if I'm resilient." He began to use the Essential Principles of Resilience he himself had laid out, including optimism, cognitive flexibility, finding a role model, and facing fear. He began positive self-talk right away. Finding a role model was also easy. He told me the POWs he had studied became his role models. "I figured if one of these guys could be a POW for eight years, then maybe I could overcome this."

Then he moved into the other elements, including actively using coping skills, having a social support network, developing emotional intelligence, and recognizing strengths. "First, I set goals for myself," he told me. He knew, from his decades of research on what helps people overcome trauma, that goal setting is a key coping mechanism. Finding something to work toward also meant focusing on strengths, and building from them. For Charney, his goal was to be able to deliver the dean's address at the annual White Coat ceremony for incoming medical students. The ceremony was in two weeks. This motivated him to work hard—despite the pain—at his physical therapy sessions, where the Bruce Springsteen song "Tougher Than the Rest" kept playing in his mind. It became his personal "fight song." He stayed focused on making it out of the ICU and back to his students at Mount Sinai.

And he did make it. When he took the stage, just two weeks after an attempt on his life, he was greeted with a standing ovation. He told his students to be prepared to face loss and disappointment daily, but to not give up. He stood before them, an example of resilience in action. He told me that while he was recovering, the students created an award in his honor—the Dean Charney Award for Resilience. "Hands down," he told me, "it's the best award I've ever gotten."

Since his own experience with trauma, Charney's passion and purpose has focused on making resilience training accessible and available—especially to the staff at Mount Sinai Hospital, which was ground zero during the COVID pandemic. During that time, Charney watched in awe as his frontline staff—especially nurses—embraced their commitment to healing, working with the sick and dying before the nature of the virus was clearly understood. These first responders worked fourteen-hour days and were often the only person present when a COVID victim was dying. They had to step in and be the human link between quarantined patients and their anxious, fearful loved ones, who had to say goodbye over a cell phone held up by a gloved and masked healthcare worker. These medical professionals worked tirelessly, despite the high risk to their own health, their time away from family, and the unremitting stress around the virus. In other words, Charney watched his colleagues navigate their way through the trauma of the early days of the pandemic with bravery, commitment, compassion, and professionalism.

In response to this and anticipating the PTSD they would suffer in the wake of the pandemic, he and his colleagues created the Mount

The Origins of the Resilience Response

Sinai Center for Stress, Resilience and Personal Growth, a multidisciplinary center to offer resilience training, mental- and physical-health services, and other vital support to the frontline healthcare providers and other staff, faculty, and students at Mount Sinai. Building from Charney's research and experience, the program was designed to address the emotional, mental, physical, and spiritual needs of the community to prevent the onset of mental health issues by virtue of early intervention, treatment, and training in building resilience.

What Charney's story illustrates, and what resilience researchers and theorists over the last several decades have all come to understand, is that resilience is within us and accessible to all of us. All it takes is the right kind of support to activate it. Psychologist Ann Masten, of the Institute of Child Development at the University of Minnesota, describes this as "ordinary magic," which she defines as being in the right environment, with the right relationships, and the right opportunities. When these systems are in place, a child can safely get to know herself and test out how best to respond to the world around her. When a child has access to the health-promoting resources, she will be able to meet life's challenges with confidence, flexibility, and acceptance. Masten's ordinary magic is all around us—if we know where to look for it.

That said, it's important to recognize that it can be harder for some of us to tap into our innate resilience because of odds stacked against us: There are inequities built even into our health system, which reflect even deeper ones in our society at large. It's easy to tell someone to eat healthier, less processed foods and get regular exercise; it's much harder to put these habits into practice if you live in poverty in an urban food desert where affordable, healthy foods are hard to come by, and where you fear for your safety should you try to take a daily walk in your neighborhood. Within the healthcare system, clinical research has long focused on the white male, excluding women and people of color from even being the subjects of study. And the medical experiences of women and minorities are not only understudied or overlooked; often people from these groups are more likely to be misdiagnosed, have their symptoms dismissed, and receive less aggressive treatment than white males. For example, a study published in the *Journal of the American Heart Association* found that women were less likely than men to receive timely treatment for heart attacks, even when they presented with the same symptoms. Another study, published in *JAMA Network Open*, found that Black patients were more likely than white patients to be diagnosed with a mental health condition even when they presented with the same physical symptoms.

Julie Palmer, director of the Slone Epidemiology Center at Boston University and founding leader of the Black Women's Health Study, which has followed fifty-nine thousand African American women since 1995, says racism and other stressors may be much stronger predictors of poor health than individual choices or genetic differences. "Structural racism affects where people live, how they can exercise, the foods they eat, and the resources available to them," she notes. The psychological trauma of racial discrimination may also increase cortisol (the body's stress hormone) and weaken the immune system, with links to elevated blood pressure, memory problems, and other conditions.

Despite enormous hurdles presented by structural inequities and racism, resilience psychology nevertheless resoundingly points to the availability of resilience to all of us, regardless of the traumas, challenges, and failures we face. Yet understanding how it affects health outcomes, and vice versa, is a new frontier in theory and research, and one that I'll explore in the next chapter. And that begins with a discussion about stress, and how we manage it.

CHAPTER 2

Why Stress Is the Heart of the Matter

Year after year, the American Heart Association reports that cardiovascular disease (CVD) is the leading cause of death for people of all genders in the United States—and worldwide. Every thirty-four seconds in the United States a person dies from cardiovascular disease. The figures are astounding, enough to stop you in your tracks. And then the questions begin: Why? What can we do? How can we stop this?

As strange and counterintuitive as it sounds, what I appreciate about CVD, and why I devoted my life to understanding and treating it, is how much we can do to prevent, combat, and reverse it. As opposed to many other medical diseases and conditions, you can guard against cardiovascular disease—and survive it. In fact, CVD is 80 percent preventable through lifestyle choices. We also have great medications, procedures, and treatments that mean there is real potential for many who suffer from CVD to fully recover and go on to live productive lives at full capacity.

On the other hand, the scary part about cardiovascular disease is that it can be so deadly—and can kill you quickly. It can go unnoticed and be silent until the day someone has a heart attack or stroke. A heart attack or stroke can happen when a stable plaque, or blockage, suddenly becomes unstable and ruptures. Or when blockages in the arteries build up severely, causing symptoms such as chest pain or shortness of breath. The electrical system of the heart can also malfunction, causing the heart to slow down, speed up, or become irregular in a way that can increase the risk of heart failure, stroke, or death. Also the cells in the heart and brain cannot regenerate, so once those cells die from a heart attack or stroke, there is no way to bring them back. The heart overall also has no backup system in the body, unlike the way we have a spare kidney or a liver that can partially regenerate.

But what seems like a dichotomy between preventability and treatability, and sudden death or major disability, in fact exists on a spectrum. And the broadest bands of the spectrum by far are on the positive, manageable side, where we can prevent and treat heart disease with things completely within our control: exercise, nutrition (we'll discuss those in a later chapter), and how to manage stress.

What Is Stress?

In physics, stress refers to the interaction between a force and a resistance to counter that force. This technical definition certainly seems to resonate with feelings we all have seemingly daily: Modern life seems to create constant obstacles to whatever we try to accomplish, ranging from the mundane (being stuck in traffic) to the shattering (the unexpected loss of a loved one).

And these feelings we experience in our minds have a real and measurable impact on the body. That's how stress has increasingly become a health problem, for more and more of the population. The American Heart Association notes several studies that make the point that "most forms of psychological distress (e.g., anger, anxiety, depression, PTSD) lead to activation of the hypothalamic-pituitary-adrenal axis, resulting in dysregulation of the autonomic nervous system and a cascade of downstream effects that can increase the risk of developing CVD." In other words, when we feel stressed, our brain signals that hormones should be released through our bloodstream, and this leads to a cascade of reactions that can directly and negatively impact heart health.

It's important to note that stress is not inherently bad; in fact, a degree of stress is required for meeting life's challenges. For example, when we're confronted with a sudden, unexpected danger (a near-miss car accident, for example), our brain registers this potential harm and triggers a series of neuroendocrine events that prepare us to either freeze, fight, or flee. This spontaneous physiological response begins with the amygdala, which is part of the limbic system, a complex network of structures in the brain associated with emotions, memory, and learning. This is where sensory information is evaluated and integrated, and it is here that a potential "threat" to our safety is registered. The amygdala then relays this information, via a network of neural pathways and neurotransmitters, to the hypothalamus, a part of the brain involved in maintaining homeostasis and regulating various autonomic systems such as temperature, circadian rhythms, hunger, and thirst. When we're subjected to stress, the hypothalamus triggers a release of hormones in response. One such hormone is called corticotropin-releasing hormone, or CRH. This chemical messenger activates what scientists refer to as the hypothalamic-pituitary-adrenocortical axis (the HPA axis), a complex communication system that connects the central nervous system and the endocrine system. The pituitary gland, another key component of the endocrine system, then releases adrenocorticotropic hormone into the bloodstream, and when this reaches your adrenal glands, they, in turn, release multiple hormones, including cortisol, which is considered one of the most important of all stress-related hormones.

We all know what this cascade of hormones feels like: We become more alert as our heart rate goes up and we send more oxygen to the brain; all of our senses suddenly become heightened. We call it an adrenaline rush. When cortisol is released, it triggers the release of glucose (blood sugar) and fat, both vital sources of energy that we will need to respond to perceived danger.

While our neuroendocrine system is ratcheting up, other systems and processes slow, including our digestive and reproductive systems. Our growth hormones become muted as well, as every available resource goes toward preparing the body to respond to the immediate threat.

All of this occurs instantaneously. Now, with the amygdala and the hypothalamus working in concert, and with the prompted cascade of hormones energizing the body to ensure our physical survival, we act; we jump out of the crosswalk and back onto the curb just before the speeding car runs the red light and hits us. Once out of danger, our nervous system sends an "all clear" message to our brain, and our body stops releasing the hormones we needed to survive this threat. In short order, our internal systems calm down and return to a regulated balance, or homeostasis. The stress came, we conquered, and now we can calmly move on. That's what we think of as acute stress.

But something very different happens to us—both psychologically and physically—when our brain perceives a threat that, for one reason or another, doesn't seem to pass. This is when stress becomes chronic. Chronic stress takes a terrible toll on our mental and physical health.

One of my favorite books that explores acute versus chronic stress is the aptly titled *Why Zebras Don't Get Ulcers* by renowned primatologist Robert Sapolsky. In it he asks why animals can engage a useful stress response that helps with survival, where in humans the signal sometimes gets scrambled: We experience stress triggered by events that are not truly threatening, and we tend to stay hypervigilant even long after any danger (real or perceived) has passed. As he notes, "A zebra's stress response kicks in when the zebra is chased by a lion: when the zebra escapes, the stress response shuts off. In between predation attempts the zebra is at ease. It doesn't flood itself with stress hormones wondering when the next lion is going to show up." We humans, on the other hand, are constantly looking around the corner for the next lion or are haunted by the ones we've already evaded.

I had the chance to talk to Sapolsky, who is also a neurobiologist and professor at Stanford University, about the psychological and physiological toll of chronic stress. Sapolsky became interested in primates at a young age and has studied them throughout his career, focusing on how adaptability to stress affected their evolution. He frequently talks about how we mammals experience optimal health when we're in homeostasis, when all of our physiological systems are performing as they should (heart rate, blood pressure, glucose levels, hormones, etc. are working in concert, sure and steady). But when faced with stress, stress-hormone levels spike, prompting us to fight or flee or freeze. Sapolsky points out that this is the stress experience for 99 percent of the mammals on earth, who experience survival-driven bursts of intense physical stress, rather than experiencing long-term existential or psychological stress.

Humans, on the other hand, are prone to ongoing *psychological* stress, such as worrying about a thirty-year mortgage, or climate change, or any number of real or imagined long-term threats to our well-being that might keep us up at night. This kind of stress—which might be described as a low-grade chronic stress, relative to the powerful, intermittent bursts of stress we (and other mammals) may experience—prevents our bodies from returning to homeostasis. Chronic low-grade stress, when our bodies are constantly experiencing a stress response, is more harmful to us than the stressor itself. "If every day is an emergency, we pay a metabolic price for this," Sapolsky says. Living with this low-grade chronic stress, studies now show, taxes all kinds of bodily systems, which can eventually lead to so many of our modern chronic illnesses such as diabetes, hypertension, and coronary artery disease—the number one killer in this country. Chronic stress also leads to chronic high blood pressure, which leads to a whole host of heart ailments, none of which are entirely reversible.

I spoke with Sapolsky during the pandemic, which, as he pointed out, was a unique period of ambiguous stress that affected humans across the globe. None of us knew how long we would be social distancing, or what we, as individuals, could do to help turn the tide on the pandemic, short of washing our hands, wearing masks, getting vaccinated, and keeping a distance from our supportive social networks. We were at the mercy of this virus for an unknown period of time, and the unremitting stress this caused inevitably took a toll on all of us.

In 2025, though the pandemic is behind us, and we've moved into a "new normal," the ravages of that time are all around us: kids who fell behind academically and socially; increased rates of depression and anxiety across all age groups; adapting to a new "hybrid" work model; and more. What, Sapolsky and I wondered together during our conversation, would the cost of this unremitting stress be on our bodies and brains long term?

Stress and the Brain

It's worth taking some time to learn more about how stress can impact the brain and the heart, the two organs that are arguably the most essential for our survival and are deeply connected to each other and

Why Stress Is the Heart of the Matter

to all other organs in our body. They are the drivers of how the rest of our body reacts to and manages stress.

The brain is an astoundingly resilient organ. It is designed to take in all the stimulation the world around us provides and process it in ways that inform our thinking, our memories, and our emotions—and then to interact with that world, and the other people in it.

Scientists refer to this quality of consumption of information and reaction as plasticity, which is the brain's ability to adapt, reorganize, and form new neural connections when stimulated by information or, yes, stress.

I've been talking about stress that can have a negative impact on the body and brain, but as I mentioned above, there's stress that has a positive impact, too. For the brain thrives on being challenged. But as with all things, it's all about the quality and quantity of that stress. Stress runs the gamut of being objectively good for us to being debilitating, and the range of stress that exists between these two extremes is endless and ever-changing and unique to each of us.

Good stress, or eustress, comes with any energizing challenge that boosts our brain chemistry and sharpens our senses and fuels our desire to perform at our peak. We see this with those who excel at their chosen profession, whether they're athletes, scientists, educators, or entrepreneurs. Training for a race, tackling a new challenge at work, planning for a big event to mark a happy occasion, mastering a new piece of music on an instrument, and preparing for a performance can all be sources of eustress. When we experience eustress, our body responds in a similar way to how it responds to distress. Our heart rate increases, breathing quickens, muscles tense. But with eustress, we view the challenge as positive and motivating, leading to a sense of excitement and focus. Repeated exposure to eustress can actually strengthen our body's ability to handle stress of any kind. This is because the body learns to efficiently activate and deactivate the stress response system. Then, when we encounter a stressful situation that is not positive, our body is better prepared to handle it.

Good stress also releases the chemicals, including endorphins, that light up our brain and foster new neural connections. Good stress tends to make us more alert, flexible, and thoughtful in our responses to people and problems. Good stress also releases the chemicals that build self-esteem and our sense of ourselves as worthwhile, proficient, and capable of growth and change. When we encounter good stress—a challenging but thought-provoking conversation, a tough test that we feel we aced—we tend to feel emotionally balanced, and a light seems to shine on the positive aspects of our lives rather than on the difficulties we've still got to manage. Our physical health also benefits from our engagement with good stress: Homeostasis is reinforced, our immune system stays strong, and our cardiovascular system is able to function well. This is when we experience a feeling of well-being.

As we face more intense stress, or any ongoing stress that we feel incapable of resolving, we run the risk of wearing down these mechanisms in our brain.

Indeed, for the past fifty years, researchers have been able to see a direct link between intense or chronic stress and changes in the brain. Chronic stress can arise from such things as job insecurity or unemployment, bullying in the workplace or at school, being in a physically or mentally abusive relationship, caring for someone with an ongoing illness or disability, or social isolation or facing discrimination. This kind of stress interferes with the brain's metabolic systems, disrupting the homeostatic release of brain hormones, which in turn causes disruptions in the "downstream" release of other hormones such as adrenaline and cortisol. Under constant dysregulation, the performance and even the size and shape of some structures of the brain may be adversely altered; a decrease in volume has been seen in both an overstressed hippocampus as well as the prefrontal cortex, or the area of the brain where decision-making, emotional regulation, memory, and other processes we associate with sociability and emotional intelligence occur. The amygdala, which plays a key role in processing emotions, particularly fear and anxiety, can also be affected. All of these essential processes can be dulled or disrupted by exposure to unremitting stress. As these structures weaken, neurogenesis (the growth of new neurons) slows, and our brains weaken.

We see this damage in a host of brain-health issues, such as cognitive dysfunction, problems with memory, or potential chronic illnesses such as depression or anxiety. When we're profoundly stressed, our brain chemistry is thrown off and then our mood suffers. Our lifestyle may begin to crack and crumble; we may have trouble falling or staying asleep; we may find our diet becomes overreliant on sugars and carbs as we seek out foods that activate the brain's reward centers as a coping mechanism. However, by consciously shifting our response to stress—through practices described in this book, even—we can begin to rewire our brains, rebuild healthy habits, and reclaim control over our mental and physical well-being, effectively reversing this decline.

But nothing tries our health more dramatically than traumatic stress, the most extreme of all stressors.

It is estimated that fully half of all US adults will have at least one traumatic experience in their lifetime. However, fewer than 7 percent of these people, it is estimated, will develop what is clinically categorized as post-traumatic stress disorder, or PTSD, according to the National Center for PTSD, housed in the US Department of Veterans Affairs. The majority of people who experience a traumatic event have acute but transient stress, which manifests after the incident in reminders of the exposure. Even so, most people recover from the trauma and these aftereffects while avoiding long-term neurobiological consequences.

George Bonanno, the noted expert on trauma and resilience, wrote a book about this called *The End of Trauma: How the New Science of Resilience Is Changing How We Think About PTSD*. Bonanno's research shows that most of us can experience and process highly traumatic events without tipping into a psychologically disordered state, such as PTSD, depression, or intractable grief. We can experience a stressful event without our brain processing it in a way that would lead to its being labeled a "traumatic" event.

Bonanno found that every person responds uniquely to stress and, importantly, responds differently each time they are exposed to a new stress. His research suggests that most of us can respond resiliently to a traumatic experience, processing and integrating its meaning, and coming away hardier than we were before. Then, when we next face an extraordinarily stressful situation, we can tap into the memory of the previous event and our recollection will reassure us, "Ah. I've encountered something unexpected/daunting/fear-inducing before and I got through it, so I will get through this, too."

Bonanno and his colleagues analyzed the findings of more than fifty studies that looked at individual responses to potentially traumatizing events. These included such things as the loss of a loved one, job, or housing; the onset of a serious illness or disease; or surviving a natural disaster, such as a hurricane, among others. The data shows that fully 65 percent of people who went through these difficult experiences showed no signs of lasting traumatic injury. This finding runs counter to what we often hear, that the effect of traumatic stress is long-lasting and near impossible to overcome.

Why Stress Is the Heart of the Matter

Bonanno's work challenges that assumption. He argues that there is always an opportunity that comes with adversity, that we humans are designed to be positively tested when we encounter even the most intense stressors. He believes (and I wholeheartedly agree) that responding resiliently—before an event can be thought of or processed as traumatizing and therefore automatically harmful—offers us the opportunity to grow psychologically and heal physically. This is what Bonanno and other experts in the field refer to as the "resilience paradox."

What happens in the immediate aftermath of a potentially traumatic event has a lot to do with whether there is likely to be positive growth. Early intervention, what we call psychological first aid, can make a profound difference in mental health outcomes after trauma. This phenomenon was explored in the scientific literature as long ago as the 1950s and received a lot more attention after the events of 9/11. Psychological first aid has since been standardized, with official training programs run by institutions such as the World Health Organization and academic credentials offered by the Institute for Disaster Mental Health at SUNY. This first aid is now offered by first responders and others who help people in the wake of natural disasters, terrorism, sexual assault, and active combat, and to others at high risk for developing PTSD. One hugely important factor in the success of psychological first aid is reaching people as soon as possible after the potentially traumatic event.

Psychological first aid interventions can be psychosocial or pharmacological, or both, and the reasons they work are many and varied. But of particular interest and fascination for me are signs that early psychological interventions after trauma can inhibit some of the hormonal and genomic changes that occur in a person's brain that then make them more likely to develop PTSD. For instance, several studies have looked at the hippocampus, a brain structure affected by stress and trauma, and found a link between cognitive behavioral therapy (CBT) and increased hippocampal volume in PTSD patients. It would make sense, then, that early interventions that include CBT could help reduce the amount of damage to the hippocampus. This is just one example of one mechanism; if we could reach more people touched by trauma sooner, we could have a dramatic impact on their mental and physiological health, in both the short and long term.

One institution that conducts early interventions to help combat PTSD is Mount Sinai Hospital in New York City, one of the first and most important medical facilities to treat frontline workers in the aftermath of 9/11. After the immediate, life-threatening physical conditions were dealt with, the hospital enacted a robust mental health program with early screening and treatment in both individual and group settings for PTSD, anxiety, depression, and other conditions to help with these potentially debilitating effects. That program grew into the World Trade Center Health Program, which through a federal act that funds it, continues to this day to provide free medical monitoring, treatment, mental health services, and counseling for 9/11 responders and volunteers. It turns out that the first responders—people conducting psychological first aid included—are also more susceptible to behavioral health conditions including depression and post-traumatic stress disorder, more so than the general population by about 10 percent. The Mount Sinai program and others like it that reach people after cataclysmic events as soon as possible can help individuals maintain resilience in the face of the worst events we can possibly imagine. My own hospital system, Northwell, has a Center for Traumatic Stress, Resilience and Recovery for employees and their families, of which a key component is the Stress First Aid program. The Northwell hospital system has also been working in Ukraine to train health providers in administering stress first aid to war survivors. How people respond to stress, and how quickly they are helped in responding to it, can make a big difference in outcomes.

In some cases, though, traumatic stress results in PTSD. Again, it is the exception and not the norm for how our brain reacts to stress; as I mentioned earlier, according to the National Center for PTSD, only about six out of every one hundred people (or less than 7 percent of the US population) will have PTSD in their lifetime. But the effect this syndrome has on the brain and its structures and functionality can be devastating.

Imaging shows us that the area of the brain associated with emotions (the amygdala) becomes hyperactive when stressed over time, producing more fear and anxiety. While this is happening, the seat of memory in the brain (the hippocampus) loses volume and functions less robustly. The area that regulates our emotions (the prefrontal cortex) is also adversely impacted, which may make it difficult for us to regulate our emotions and our impulses, and this may lead to poor decision-making.

It is also important to understand why some people are more susceptible to developing PTSD when exposed to trauma than others. Research has shown that prior exposure to trauma, family psychiatric history, and lack of social support are all related to a predisposition to developing PTSD. Studies also show that approximately one-third of the vulnerability to develop PTSD is genetically inheritable. But our genetics, as Bonanno wrote, are not our destiny; this means that the other two thirds of our vulnerability to PTSD is determined by environment and experience. Also, given the genetic component, we should be able, and indeed we have begun, to identify and isolate genes that predict the development of PTSD—offering hope that we might be able to figure out who among trauma survivors is especially vulnerable to the condition. This could help us in deciding who would most likely require and respond well to early interventions, instead of their being sentenced to suffering.

Stress affects the brain in profound ways. Identifying them is the first step. We can then understand how we might disrupt those changes—by mounting a Resilience Response.

Stress and the Heart

The brain is the control center for how we respond to stress overall. But stress, as you might have guessed, also affects other key organs in the body, including the heart.

Like the brain, it thrives on a type of good stress. Think exercise. Exertion causes our heart to work harder, to build healthy muscle cells, which then make it stronger, which in turn leads to better circulation, allows an easier flow of blood through the body, which leads to clearer arteries and lower blood pressure. The US government's Office of Disease Prevention and Health Promotion (ODPHP) recommends that we each strive for 150 minutes of moderate aerobic exercise or 75 minutes of vigorous aerobic exercise per week, to promote heart health and prevent the onset of disease. The American Heart Association published a study in the journal *Circulation* in 2022 that found those who met these basic weekly exercise guidelines lowered their risk of dying by as much as 21 percent. Those who exceeded these guidelines by two to four times lowered their risk of mortality by 31 percent. What this shows us is that the more physical stress your body endures when you walk, run, play, or work out, the greater your health.

Moving your body in any way you enjoy is far, far better than being sedentary. Our bodies are designed to function optimally when they are in motion, and we know that being inactive can have serious health consequences, including promoting cardiovascular disease (as well as high

Why Stress Is the Heart of the Matter

blood pressure, cancer, and diabetes, and other preventable diseases). Because of technology, most of us spend too much time either sitting in our cars commuting or sitting at a desk staring at a screen. Our sedentary lifestyles and the causal link between inactivity and the onset of disease should prompt all of us to move more and seek out good stress.

That link was on my mind when I first met Harold, a patient referred to me at the age of fifty-seven. He'd recently begun experiencing shortness of breath whenever he'd climb stairs. In his general-health questionnaire, Harold indicated that he'd once been a pack-a-day cigarette smoker, but that he'd quit twenty years ago. He rarely drank. And he was not taking any medication, except for the occasional pain reliever. He was slightly overweight, but otherwise, he seemed to be in pretty good health. He told me that he was stressed-out at work, but otherwise he was happily married, had a couple of kids in college, and felt as if his life was, to use his words, "pretty decent." I asked him what he did for work, and he told me he was an accountant for an investment firm and that the company had recently been audited. I asked him how long he thought he sat at his desk every day. "I used to be a nine-to-fiver, but now I have to work nights and weekends, too. So I'm probably sitting for ten to twelve hours a day." He shook his head. "Maybe even longer. Sometimes I feel like I go from my desk to my bed, work is that busy." I asked him when he found time to exercise. He laughed and replied, "Never."

I decided to give him a cardiac stress test. The test, as the name implies, makes your heart work harder to see how it responds, usually by exercising on a treadmill. If you can't exercise, medication can be used to simulate exercise. Your heart's electrical activity (ECG) and blood pressure, and sometimes images of your heart (echocardiogram or nuclear scan), are monitored. While this is happening, doctors are looking for signs of ischemia—basically, that the heart muscle isn't getting enough blood. Unusual activity on the ECG or symptoms such as fatigue, shortness of breath, and chest pain might point to that. If so, the concern is that there might be blockages in the coronary arteries, which supply blood to your heart. These blockages, usually caused by plaque buildup (atherosclerosis), restrict blood flow and create symptoms. If the blockages are severe, they can also increase the risk of a heart attack.

Harold's stress test indicated that he likely had significant coronary artery disease. I next sent him for a cardiac catheterization procedure, which confirmed that he had narrowing in one of his main coronary arteries, and he ended up having a stent placed in that artery to increase the blood flow to his heart.

When we sat down after this procedure, we talked about how important lifestyle is to managing coronary disease. I asked Harold if there'd been a time when he'd been more physically active, and he told me he'd been a pretty serious athlete, having been a competitive swimmer through college. He lit up as he told me how calming, even meditative, he found the hours of intensive training to be, and how fun competing had been.

Was it possible, I asked, for him to find time to get back in the pool?

He perked up and told me there was a health club not far from his office that had a pool. I shared with him the government health office recommendation of getting 150 minutes of exercise per week (or about two and a half hours), saying that whatever he could manage to work toward this goal would really benefit his heart. He said he'd give it a try. Then he asked me if I was going to write him a prescription.

Let's see how you do with the gym first, I replied. Lifestyle change is an incredibly effective tool and sometimes negates the need for pharmacological intervention. Its power comes through helping to target and change our physiology. For instance, lifestyle change such as improving your diet, exercising, and managing your weight and your stress levels can directly combat atherosclerosis by lowering cholesterol levels, especially "bad" cholesterol or LDL, which contributes to plaque formation. It can also help lower blood pressure, basically reducing the force of blood against artery walls, and improve the health of the inner lining of blood vessels, making them more resistant to plaque formation.

We started with lifestyle changes and I scheduled a follow-up for three months later.

When I saw Harold next, he told me he had been going to the gym at lunchtime and was swimming for a half hour three days a week. This meant he was logging one and a half hours a week of exercise, which was a great start toward the recommended two and a half hours.

When I saw him again three months later, he was now swimming five days a week and had added some strength training to his workouts. He had dropped ten pounds and was sleeping better, and his energy and his mood and outlook had greatly improved.

That's how good stress affects the heart.

But acute stress can affect what we refer to as "cardiac tone," which is the contracting strength of the heart muscle. Think of a clenched fist. Now think of that clenched fist being covered and squeezed hard by another hand. That forced contraction is what stress does to cardiac tone—it strains the usual action of the muscle.

When this happens repeatedly (or when acute stress becomes chronic), it can lead to other cardiovascular issues such as high blood pressure. And this is when the dominoes begin to fall—this type of stress not only induces hypertension, but it can raise your heart rate and cause inflammation, which may in turn cause artery damage and the development of plaques, which can in turn lead to a heart attack, stroke, or other cardiovascular illnesses. Chronic stress can also influence blood clotting, further increasing the risk for these events. It also may disrupt your ability to get a good night's sleep, and a lack of sleep raises the risk of developing heart disease or worsening existing heart disease. When you're sleep-deprived, your mood plummets and you no longer have the energy to make heart-healthy lifestyle adjustments, and so your diet slips, you gain weight, you exercise less—I could go on, but the point is, the whole cycle that chronic stress triggers wreaks havoc on your cardiovascular health from every possible angle.

And it's not just your cardiovascular health, or your brain health. Stress affects your overall health in all sorts of ways.

How Stress Affects Overall Health

The establishment of modern medicine at roughly the turn of the twentieth century (which included addressing widespread public health issues such as sanitation, infectious diseases, and safety), coupled with the explosive evolution of the medical profession itself, caused a great improvement in the general health of the average American. As vaccines, antibiotics, and other medicines were discovered and used, the rate of death by infectious diseases began to decline, and the age of mortality began to rise. Over the fifty years between 1900 and 1950, the leading causes of death went from being infectious diseases such as tuberculosis, pneumonia, and influenza to being *chronic* diseases, such as heart disease, cancer, and others. And yet, by 1950, the average American life spanned sixty-eight years—an impressive increase of twenty years in only half a century.

This stunning increase in longevity gave the medical community hope that they were doing something right. But a big, complex question also came to light at this time: We could identify what was influencing the shift away from short, sharp, infectious-disease deaths, but why were rates of the often long, progressive, and ultimately fatal chronic diseases rising? What factor was driving this?

Why Stress Is the Heart of the Matter

Could it be stress?

That question has caused scientists and researchers to begin to quantitatively understand the physiological ramifications of stress. And given that we're decades into the serious study of stress, we have an answer. Yes, it's absolutely a big contributing factor (as you might have suspected from the previous sections in this chapter).

We know stress basically elicits one of two biological responses. As we've already seen, the first is a response to acute stress—the fight, flight, or freeze reaction, which hits hard and fast, then gives way to calm and balance, a restoration of homeostasis. The second is a response to chronic stress, where the fight, flight, or freeze response is ignited, but then . . . never quite goes out. When we're subjected to chronic stress, we're "on," to varying degrees, and this can take a terrible toll on the body (hence the name *chronic diseases*).

By the year 2000, the leading causes of death remained basically the same as those from 1950: heart disease, cancer, stroke, diabetes, and other chronic diseases. But now, the life expectancy in the United States had soared another eight years to an average of seventy-seven years. Why? Because although the leading causes of death remained the same, the rate of death had declined, thanks to better medical care, positive lifestyle changes . . . and our growing awareness of the toll stress takes on not just the brain and the heart, but on the whole body.

The logical conclusion to this would be that, although we now appear to be dying from chronic diseases, we're living longer, so why worry? Fair enough. But if you take another look at the average age of death in the United States over the intervening years, a stress-inducing (sorry) trend emerges. Since 2000, there have, of course, been minor fluctuations in US life expectancy averages. Over this roughly quarter-century span, average life expectancy in the United States peaked in 2014 at 78.9, according to the CDC's National Center for Health Statistics. In 2023, it had declined to 77.5 years—that's a big plunge in under a decade.

In a *Washington Post* podcast that aired in early 2023, Dean Michelle Williams and Professor Asaf Bitton, MD, from the Chan School of Public Health at Harvard University sounded the alarm about this plunge. But what they both pointed to as the cause of this alarming statistic took me by surprise.

"We have a wonderful sick-care system that takes care of very sick people, but a very inadequate healthcare system," said Bitton. He separated our system into these two parts.

This is because, as these two public health experts know too well, our healthcare system is wholly oriented toward treating the very sick, including the chronically ill, at the expense of disease prevention. That is particularly true when it comes to diseases associated with chronic stress.

One fascinating and important concept when it comes to understanding chronic stress and what it does to our bodies and our minds is that of allostatic load. We know that homeostasis is what our systems seek: a state of stability. Allostasis is the process by which the body responds to stressors to try to regain that state.

Allostatic load, in turn, refers to the cumulative and combined burden of chronic stress and life events. It's the wear and tear our bodies sustain. Allostatic load is not just a psychological concept; it can be measured with biomarkers and clinical criteria.

When it all gets too much, then allostatic overload ensues. This can result in impaired health and even reduced longevity. Low socioeconomic status is associated with high allostatic load, as people who are struggling to make ends meet or who live in poverty are more likely to experience higher degrees of chronic stress than people of a higher socioeconomic status. One multilevel analysis done using survey data from Detroit, Michigan, combined with the 2000 US Census conclusively found that neighborhood poverty in the city was positively associated with allostatic load. Other studies have revealed similar findings—and even more granular ones, such as linking allostatic load to an increased incidence of type 2 diabetes or coronary heart disease in neighborhoods where poverty is endemic.

The deep-seated inequities woven into our society mean certain groups of people deal with a baseline level of stress that others do not have to account for. In the 1990s, Dr. Arline Geronimus, a public health researcher and professor of health behavior and health education at the University of Michigan, proposed the "weathering hypothesis" to describe the negative and cumulative effects of chronic stress on the physical and mental health of the politically and societally marginalized. She gathered data on more than three hundred thousand pregnant women to understand the racial disparities in infant mortality rates. Black teen mothers, she discovered, were giving birth to healthier babies than their older counterparts, and she postulated that this was because they had endured fewer years of discrimination (chronic stress) than even mothers of color in their twenties. Her thesis was ridiculed, with accusations made that she was promoting teen pregnancy. Calls were made for Michigan to fire her (the university wisely declined). She got death threats.

But thirty years later, cross-disciplinary research supports Geronimus's work. Now it's being celebrated for providing a framework to study the health consequences caused by the stress of social inequity.

In 2023, Geronimus published *Weathering: The Extraordinary Stress of Ordinary Life in an Unjust Society*, which eloquently articulates how, regardless of race, living without political representation or social or economic capital leads to chronic illness and premature death. In the "weathering" she and other researchers describe, the body breaks down over prolonged exposure to the chronic environmental stressors caused by inequality. These societal stressors, which often persist over generations, leave people vulnerable to poverty, crime, and the kinds of chronic stress that ultimately lead to the onset of chronic diseases such as obesity, diabetes, and cardiovascular illnesses. It's nearly impossible for people who live under these circumstances to tap into the resources they need to build resilience, and this has created an ongoing public health crisis. The only way to address this is with vast, systemic cultural and political change, including a sea change in how our medical system incorporates our understanding of societal stress and inequity into the ways we practice healthcare.

That will not happen suddenly or soon. And it's not fair. But unfortunately, in the meantime it is imperative that we learn to identify, manage, and *live with* stress; it's not about overcoming, it's about transforming our response to it. It isn't always easy to mount such a response, especially for those living in marginalized or disadvantaged communities.

People need resources to help them figure out how to handle stress to live well, and to live longer. And it's not something our healthcare system is built to teach.

I've learned that there is no way I can adequately treat my patients if I don't get to know them and their surrounding life circumstances and understand what kind of stress they are under. And the latter, though they aren't the kind of thing that we can easily test for, are essential to know about and understand if I'm going to be able to truly help people. The only way to find out what kind of stress a person is dealing with is to ask. And then to listen. To really listen.

I was reminded of that crucial fact when I met Mary. Mary came to me with high blood pressure. She was in her early forties, though she looked considerably older. She told me she was working two jobs to support her family. Her husband was injured on a construction job and couldn't work at the time. Mary had three kids, all still at home with her. When we first met, Mary told me that she'd been a smoker since the age of eighteen. She sheepishly explained that she knew how bad it was for her, but that quitting was just something she had not been able to do.

So I asked her, "How do you think smoking has helped you?"

This question took her completely by surprise. "It just calms my nerves," she told me. "John's been out of work for a year now. I feel like I can barely hold our household together, you know?" I nodded and let her continue. "Believe it or not, a smoke break seems to be the only time I can either step away from work or step outside of our house and have a moment to myself."

What I heard was that, for nearly thirty years, smoking was a reliable, effective source of stress relief and even comfort to Mary. It helped, she went on, to ground her. She's an informed person, and she already knew that the risks to her health far outweighed the comfort from smoking. So instead of pressing her on the obvious need for her to quit, I focused on her need for meaningful comfort and support.

Mary told me that no one in her life had asked her what she might need to feel less stressed, less burdened by so much responsibility. It wasn't that her husband and children didn't care about her, it just never dawned on her to ask them for support. Especially since her husband's accident, Mary had positioned herself as the "strong one," the person to absorb the stresses of life on behalf of the rest of the family. But her style of coping—and her determination to manage her family's stress all on her own—was no longer serving her. It was wearing her down. And that day in my office, she was beginning to accept that her inadequate coping skills were at a cost to her health. This was a profound moment of self-awareness for her. And we were now engaged in an important, intimate conversation about her life.

The Healing Power of Resilience

I suggested she might want to try different strategies for coping. Could she, perhaps, ask her husband to prepare a few meals a week or take on the task of making sure the children got their homework done so she could have some time to take care of herself? Could her children, who were between nine and twelve years of age, take on some of the housework? And when she was at work, could she use the few minutes she took for her smoke breaks for mini-health-breaks instead? For example, instead of lighting up, could she do some deep breathing? Drink some water? Take a brisk walk around the block? Listen to a five-minute meditation? We started to brainstorm together. Until she'd come into my office, she'd been so head down, just trying to get by day-to-day, she hadn't allowed herself the time to think about other ways she might respond to stress.

While we discussed the importance of her ultimately quitting smoking, I made the conscious decision to encourage Mary to focus not on what she shouldn't do, but on what she could do. I knew that if I got her to focus on what she could change (her own behavior) as opposed to what she could not (her husband's currently being unable to work), she would draw upon her own sense of agency, and this would help her navigate the very real stressors she had to contend with.

And she did. As Mary proved, we can learn to have a different relationship to stress to ultimately prevent or slow the onset of cardiovascular and other diseases it can cause. That's what the Resilience Response is all about.

One of the ultimate stressors, both acute and chronic, can be health issues themselves. Receiving and dealing with a challenging diagnosis can cause our bodies to respond with both an acute and a chronic stress response. This book hopes to equip someone who may be facing a new diagnosis with mindsets and tools to help.

CHAPTER 3

Accept Your Current Situation

The Resilience Response begins with acceptance.

That might sound like an easy task—but ask anyone who has faced a trauma, a challenge, or a failure and has had to accept a new reality after, and they will tell you it is anything but easy. These moments can undo us, but they can also transform us.

I see this every day in my practice, taking care of people's heart health.

Consider this: One of the challenges of treating heart disease is that it often comes with few or no symptoms. This is why it is called the silent killer. Often, the buildup of plaque in the arteries takes years, even decades, before showing any hints that something is awry in the cardiovascular system. Sadly, a heart attack is often the first indicator of heart disease, and this kind of serious event puts the heart muscle, itself, at risk of permanent injury.

Additionally, the symptoms of heart disease (or even heart attack) are often misdiagnosed. They may mimic the symptoms of other conditions such as heartburn or indigestion or generalized fatigue. Or the symptoms may present differently in women. Rather than having crushing chest pain, for example, a woman experiencing a heart attack may present with dizziness or nausea, shortness of breath, extreme fatigue, or a pain in the shoulders, neck, or jaw. The vague discomfort a female heart attack sufferer experiences might, even now, be written off as a psychological, rather than a cardiac, problem. Readers, do not ignore these signs. Please seek out a doctor who can appropriately evaluate you. I always tell my patients it's better to make sure it's not your heart before we label it or diagnose it as something else.

But whether in males or females, cardiac health issues are often undetected until there is significant or advanced disease. Many come to the hospital not knowing how far it has progressed, and how much damage this event has done. It redirects the course of a life in an instant. To imagine what comes next, patients must both accept what often feels like a surprise diagnosis and accept the changes that diagnosis brings to their daily experience of life. That can mean medication such as statins to lower cholesterol, or anticoagulants to prevent blood clots, or beta-blockers, which slow down the heart rate and lower blood pressure, reducing the heart's workload. All of these medications have potential side effects, ranging from muscle aches to fatigue to nausea to headaches. Lifestyle changes are almost always in order as well.

Even then, I sometimes see people who do everything within their power to improve their heart health, and yet . . . their condition does not improve, or even worsens. In these cases, especially, being resilient means accepting that reality.

Sometimes, medical treatments and interventions don't work. Sometimes, they work for a time before faltering. I've treated patients who have little chance of surviving their illnesses, and sadly, but understandably, some of these patients give up and withdraw from life. Others seem to embrace the reality of their situation and recommit to living as fully as possible, maximizing the time they have left. Acceptance may not change the outcome, but it can change the daily experience of life for patients.

The hard truth is that we are all going to die. But until that day comes, we all have the chance to live our lives with purpose, meaning, and joy.

For those facing an incurable disease, this kind of acceptance can be hard, especially in our culture, where we're expected to "battle" or "fight" disease until the bitter end. But what if there is another way? What would it look like if, rather than rail against a chronic or even terminal illness, we accepted it as a new facet of who we are?

That's what happened to a patient of mine named Gary, a successful broker in his early sixties. He was referred to me when his general practitioner heard a disconcerting murmur while listening to his heart. I did a battery of tests, including an echocardiogram, and they revealed that two of Gary's four heart valves were malfunctioning significantly enough that I recommended he see a cardiac surgeon immediately. Gary was initially confused by the diagnosis, as he came to me completely asymptomatic. But when I walked him through his tests results and he was able to "see" his valve behavior on the imaging, he wasted no time. He was scheduled for surgery within the month.

Even though Gary was walked through what the surgery and his recovery would look like, he told me in our follow-up meeting six months after his procedure that the reality of the recovery took him by surprise. First, there was a complication when, just two days after surgery, his heartbeat became irregular enough that he was cardioverted—essentially, when a machine is used to deliver an electric shock to the heart to try to restore a regular rhythm. This made him acutely aware of his inherent fragility. Though he was in good shape when he went into surgery, even tasks such as getting himself to the bathroom or dressing were initially difficult for him afterward. This became, for him, important lessons in patience. Every facet of his life, he found, had been affected by this experience, and the acceptance of all of it—the diagnosis, the surgery, the recovery—had a powerful impact on him.

He told me that he was now far less quick to judge not only others, but himself. He told me that in moments when he'd otherwise get annoyed or angry, he'd stop and recall the image of his damaged valves from that original echocardiogram. When I asked him why he did this, he said the memory of those images kept him in touch with the knowledge of how precious and fleeting life is. "I took my body for granted before—especially my heart. Accepting that it's fallible has totally changed my outlook on life for the better. Now I let stuff that used to bother me slide. I want to put all my energy focusing on the good stuff, you know?"

And this isn't just a key part of preparing for, and recovering from, heart surgery. I often see patients diagnosed with atherosclerosis, the condition I described in the last chapter, grapple with acceptance. Many of these patients are shocked, as outwardly they seem to be living generally healthy lives; they are in shape, getting exercise, are a normal weight, and can't believe they could have heart disease. It is also hard for them to understand that this is not curable. Atherosclerosis can be managed, but it cannot be removed or fully reversed. They will be living with it for the rest of their life and will always be monitored or treated for this new chronic condition of coronary artery disease. And managing atherosclerosis is crucial to preventing a heart attack or stroke.

Plaque in arteries is caused by many things that we have a degree of control over (and sometimes things we don't, such as genetics or age), and that's why it is so important that I support my patients—without judgment—while they learn about the reality of their condition, including that they may have made lifestyle choices in the past (smoking, eating an excess of processed foods, being sedentary) that contributed to the development of the disease. Once they accept the fact of the disease, then we can move forward together and make a meaningful plan to slow its progression and hopefully prevent an event such as a heart attack or stroke.

The good news is that much of the cardiovascular disease I describe above can, especially if it is detected early, be managed in ways that allow us to continue to live full, active, and rich lives—but it all begins with acceptance. And acceptance means not only accepting the things we cannot change, but having the willingness *to change the things we can*.

Studies of elderly adults with arthritis, hypertension, and hearing and other impairments, patients with HIV/AIDS, patients with kidney disease who are on dialysis, and other people suffering from chronic conditions have all been shown to have more positive clinical health outcomes when they have some kind of acceptance intervention as part of their treatment. The goal is to acknowledge the illness, the limitations it may bring, and the emotional distress it may cause, without judgment or resistance. These interventions often use acceptance and commitment therapy (ACT), which can help us recognize thoughts about our illness—such as "Why me?" or "I can't do anything anymore"—and acknowledge these thoughts as just thoughts, not facts. This can reduce the power of these thoughts to cause distress. Mindfulness practices, such as meditation or deep breathing, are also powerful tools in this intervention—which is promising news for how we can practice a Resilience Response, even in the face of great challenges.

I learned my own lesson in acceptance when I had to come to terms with a health issue—thankfully not life-threatening, but potentially life-altering—while I was still studying to become a doctor. Medical school is tough, but I loved the pressure of it all, and I loved my studies. I was thriving as a student at USC. But during my sophomore year, while I was sitting in a lecture hall, something strange happened.

Once the professor dimmed the lights, flashes of colored light filled my right eye. I had always been myopic—I've worn glasses since the age of five—but this was like nothing I'd ever experienced before. It was as though a tiny firework had exploded in my eye. I went to my ophthalmologist, who saw a hemorrhage in that eye. He then sent me to a retina specialist. My retina, apparently, looked fine, but he sent me to a neuro-ophthalmologist, who administered a visual-field test. I failed it.

"You have an inferior arcuate defect," he told me.

I no longer had any vision across the bottom third of my right eye. What had caused this damage to my sight?

He speculated that I might be suffering from optic neuritis, which is often associated with MS (multiple sclerosis). Or, he casually said, perhaps I'd had some kind of stroke.

Now I was terrified. Since he had no idea what had caused my vision loss, he prescribed both a brain and spinal MRI, and the hours I spent during these tests were the most harrowing of my young life. Yet even these imaging tests did not turn up any cause for my vision loss.

When I returned to school after a holiday break, I saw another neurologist, who, mercifully, ruled out MS—for the moment. Then I saw two additional neuro-ophthalmologists, neither of whom could offer any insight into what had damaged my eye. The only consensus I got was that I should have a brain MRI every year for the next five years to continue to rule out MS. I did not find this reassuring. Not knowing what had caused this deficit in my eye left me extremely afraid: I'd go to bed at night wondering if I'd wake up with more vision loss or, worse, that I'd wake up blind. Taking a watch-and-wait approach, and the uncertainty of it all, left me even more anxious. Was my career in jeopardy? Would I lose my ability to jog, to drive? On top of all of these daily ruminations, I was in a toxic relationship with a man back where I grew up in Florida, someone who was a full decade older than I and who was putting incredible pressure on me to leave California and "come home." It was all becoming too much.

By the end of my sophomore year, I was a wreck. I didn't know if I'd be able to get through the next two years of medical school. When I got home to Florida for a brief break, I fell apart.

This is when my mother reminded me of the short prayer that she had set her life by:

God, grant me the serenity to accept the things I cannot change, the courage to change the things I can, and the wisdom to know the difference.

At the time neither my mother nor I knew this as the Serenity Prayer, the bedrock of twelve-step recovery programs. We simply knew it as the prayer my mother had latched on to when she was just a child, following the shocking, untimely death of her beloved younger sister. It had become, for both my mother and me, a prayer that reminded us of our resilience; it reminded us to accept the reality of whatever situation we faced, and then to be flexible as we set a course of action that would allow us to achieve our dreams, or simply get through, despite our losses.

My mom reminded me that I had no control over what had happened and that worrying about what hadn't happened yet would not help me meet my goal of becoming a doctor. "Don't waste your time worrying about something that might not ever happen. Just get on with your mission," she said. "Life is not perfect. And you don't have to be perfect. Just get on with your mission. Fulfill your purpose."

This one conversation with my mother shifted something within me. I was able, for the first time in six months, to see a path forward that felt empowering. I had a choice to make: I could accept what had happened and figure out a new way forward, or I could give up and remain paralyzed by the fear and the what-ifs. I knew, from that moment on, I would never give up.

My vision did not improve. But fortunately, it did not deteriorate further. To accept my new reality and succeed in medical school, I needed to refind my purpose and put my focus squarely on what fueled my desire to become a doctor in the first place: caring for other people. By doing this—by focusing on being of service to others and not allowing myself to focus on what I'd lost or what I might lose in the future—I was able to move through the anxiety and depression that had briefly stopped me, tap into my resilience, and finish medical school strong.

There is not a day that goes by that I am not aware that in an instant I could once again be a patient. Along with my white coat, I forever carry my mark of illness in my visual-field loss. That feeling of a patient's fear resides on the edge of my awareness, far enough away that I function but close enough to bring empathy. Life as a patient alters your perspective; you become a survivor. Some define a survivor as one who conquers and overcomes a disease, but I have learned to embrace a different meaning. To me, a survivor personifies the Serenity Prayer: acceptance, courage, and wisdom. My experience showed me life cannot be tamed. Rather, it is gloriously chaotic and the way to flourish is to handle the events that befall us with grace. I have learned to live with both the imperfection and the perfection in my life.

Learning How to Accept a Medical Diagnosis

Other doctors have been patients, too. In a 2016 TEDx Talk, Steven Hayes, an American psychologist renowned for his work in psychological flexibility, recounts his own early struggles with a severe panic disorder. During one particularly harrowing panic attack, alone and completely debilitated, he reached a breaking point and found himself making a profound declaration to his panic. Anguished, he shouted out, "I will not run from me!" From that moment on, he began learning to accept his pain and suffering, and over time he began to see how this process could give life meaning.

It might not surprise you to hear that he has spent the ensuing decades developing acceptance and commitment therapy. ACT combines aspects of CBT (cognitive behavioral therapy) and mindfulness in an incredibly effective way that helps those who suffer from stress-inducing conditions such as anxiety, depression, and substance abuse find relief and recovery. Both ACT and CBT emphasize the importance of changing behavior to improve outcomes. They utilize techniques such as goal setting, behavior activation, and exposure therapy to help people modify their actions and responses. ACT in particular focuses on nonjudgmental observation and acceptance of thoughts and feelings, rather than trying to control or eliminate them. This acceptance fosters a more open and nonjudgmental reflective attitude, which has been proven to lead to lower levels of distress and an increase in psychological flexibility.

In 2020, researchers specifically studied the efficacy of ACT in 12,477 participants. They found that ACT, and the acceptance it promoted, was effective in reducing anxiety, depression, substance use, and chronic pain, no matter the illness—and that included in people with multiple diagnoses. And this study is just part of a vast body of research that confirms the efficacy of ACT, for people as far ranging as parents of children with chronic conditions to heathcare workers reporting distress in clinical settings.

Another study gave evidence of how crucial this therapy can be. It focused on chronically ill adolescents and their relationship with their diseases. Out of their conclusions, the researchers developed a four-pronged

The Healing Power of Resilience

pathway toward acceptance: understanding of illness, overcoming limitations, normalization, and, finally, readiness for responsibility. They learned that patients who followed the four steps of acceptance were able to effect positive outcomes, such as improved self-esteem, increased quality of life, stronger identity, and better disease control. Patients who did not, on the other hand, experienced psychological distress.

So it's not just that acceptance can be psychologically beneficial—but it can help the patient literally get better, too. That's why I believe it's so important to a successful Resilience Response. I've seen it in my practice, and beyond.

Though I am a cardiologist, my interest extends far beyond a single organ or disease. That's what led me to become a medical correspondent for national news networks.

I interviewed a woman named Paige for a segment on the alarming uptick in late-stage breast cancer in women under forty. At only twenty-six, Paige was diagnosed with stage 2 breast cancer. She underwent chemotherapy, then a mastectomy, followed by radiation. Her treatment worked and she was given the all clear. For three years, she enjoyed being in remission. Then, at age thirty, she landed her dream job as a beauty editor at *Allure* magazine. She was also newly engaged to be married. Everything pointed to a bright future for her. But then she started experiencing hip pain. When she went to get it checked out, she was told that the cause of her pain was tumors—her breast cancer had returned and was now stage 4, having metastasized to her bone. She shared this part of her story with me calmly, holding my gaze as she spoke. "I'd be lying if I said it was easy, but positivity has always been my shield," she said.

I asked her how she was coping with this tough news, and she shared that her oncologist had suggested she think of her life as a book and that this was just the next chapter. She became thoughtful and added,

"Hopefully, this will be a very long chapter. If I need to turn a page and try a new treatment and start a new chapter, I will. But this is where I am in the story of my life, and I'm determined to live it to its fullest."

Throughout our conversation, Paige referred to herself as a "thriver," rather than a "survivor," exemplifying to me how she was meeting her diagnosis with a resilient mindset. She was accepting that cancer was now a part of her life, not something she had moved past. Finally, I asked her if there was any advice she'd gotten from her doctor that had helped her maintain this mindset. "Yes." She smiled. "He said two words: *celebrate life*. And that's exactly what I intend to do."

Paige had accepted the news of her cancer's pernicious return without it diminishing the richness of her life—her exciting job, her upcoming wedding. It was an incredible example of the Resilience Response. She accepted the reality of her situation and recommitted to living as fully as possible, maximizing the time she has left.

Looking Beyond a Medical Diagnosis

Throughout this book, I draw on examples from medicine and beyond to illustrate why the Resilience Response matters so much. My goal is to show how it can provide a blueprint to cope with many of life's stressors, whether that's a medical diagnosis or, as Dr. Lucy Hone experienced, another kind of devastating event.

Dr. Lucy Hone is a world-renowned resilience expert and psychologist. In her 2019 Ted Talk "Three Secrets of Resilient People," she begins with a series of questions: "If you've ever lost someone you truly loved, ever had your heart broken, ever struggled through an acrimonious divorce . . . please stand up." Many members of the audience rise. She continues and asks another series of far-ranging questions such as "Have you survived a natural disaster, been bullied, lost a job, had to cope with mental illness or physical impairment?" Within thirty seconds of beginning her talk, nearly the entire audience is standing. She then asks the audience to look at the room and says, simply, "Look around you. Adversity doesn't discriminate."

What Dr. Hone was showing us is that every one of us will experience heartbreak, adversity, and loss during our lifetime. She herself knows this only too intimately, through a loss that challenged everything she had learned and taught about resilience over the years.

In 2014, during a holiday weekend, her twelve-year-old daughter, Abi, was in a car with her best friend, Ella, and Ella's mother, Sally. Sally, a close friend of Dr. Hone's, was driving. A car sped through a stop sign, crashing into them and killing all three of them instantly. In that instant, Dr. Hone's world was shattered.

The people who were sent out to counsel the Hone family after the tragedy told them that they were now prime candidates for divorce, mental illness, and a whole host of other problems. Well-meaning experts shared the five stages of grief (anger, bargaining, denial, depression, and acceptance) and told the family they could pretty much write off the next five years as lost to overwhelming grief. Every message the family was given emphasized that they were now victims of this awful tragedy.

But what she needed, Dr. Hone shares, was to figure out how to be, as she says in her Ted Talk, an "active participant in my own grief process." Passively waiting for the five stages of grief to wash over her would not, she knew, heal her. Instead she put everything she'd learned from her decade of studying resilience research into action: She had to figure out how to survive this loss and be there for her husband and her two sons and continue to be a productive member of her community.

Accept Your Current Situation

Dr. Hone developed three resilience strategies that she used to navigate her way through her crushing grief. The first is that resilient people know that everyone suffers at some point in life. They know that tragedy does not discriminate and rather than lamenting "Why me?" they understand that they are as susceptible to loss as anyone else. Second, resilient people are good at choosing where they put their attention. They approach their situation with a baseline level of rational clarity, which allows them to actively pursue their healing, to adjust and course-correct so they may appropriately incorporate their loss into their lives, without being swallowed up by it. Finally, resilient people ask themselves, "Is what I'm doing helping or harming me?" They make conscious choices to engage in thoughts and behaviors that are positive and forward oriented, not destructive, self-defeating, or ruminative. For Hone, this meant asking herself if attending the trial of the driver who killed her daughter would be beneficial to her. She decided it would not be. She also realized that looking at photos of Abi often left her feeling depleted, so she stopped doing this, knowing it wasn't helping her to heal and move forward.

Each of Dr. Hone's three resilience strategies depends first on accepting a new reality. That this new reality exists is incredibly challenging to confront, but if we are to continue on in life, we must.

I had the chance to interview Dr. Hone for CBS News a couple of years ago; we talked about these strategies and more. As she put it, "I think there are quite a lot of myths about resilience in our society. I think, sadly, a lot of people think of it as some kind of elusive trait, you know, or even a fixed trait that some people have and other people don't. And that's such a shame, because actually resilience is really an amalgam of ways of thinking and acting, a whole load of different strengths and abilities and connections. And it is really available to us all, you know? There are ways of thinking and acting that can really help us navigate tough times." She underlined again that the research shows that the majority of people are resilient.

That said, there will come a moment when all the assumptions we've made about our lives, and how they'll continue to unfold, fall away. When our life is in tatters, we must make a conscious decision: Do I look backward and desperately try to stitch together that which has been torn to shreds? Or do I accept reality and accept that my assumptions about how life should be must change? Do I let go of the expectations I've held on to, for myself and others, as being no longer valid or helpful? Dr. Hone describes working through this thought process as being willing to "move the goalposts" we've had our sights set on. In our conversation she summarized this by saying, "Okay, so we're now going down that route. Didn't see that coming. Up we go, you know? Pick up your bags and off you go."

And it's not just goalposts that can move. When we've suffered a catastrophic loss, our very identity is often thrown into crisis. When Abi died, Dr. Hone had to make the conscious decision to focus on being a wife and the mother of two living boys, and to resist becoming mired in the identity of the grieving mother who had lost her daughter. She had to be present and available to her husband and sons, whose lives were also permanently altered by Abi's death. She had to figure out how to allow herself to be changed by this awful experience. Accepting that she would never be the same again was crucial to her being able to overcome her grief enough to live again.

She made the conscious decision to try out what she'd learned as a resilience expert to help her work through her own grief. Dr. Hone speaks eloquently about this in what she calls having a "co-destiny" with her daughter, even though she is gone. Dr. Hone describes creating a legacy around those who have died, to really understand how your lives

Accept Your Current Situation

have changed because of them. "So my co-destiny with Abi," she said, "is that all of the writing and speaking that I do, all the work that we do around resilient grieving, the ways of acting to help you cope with loss, it's a co-destiny because even though she's not here, I would never be doing this work without her." For Dr. Hone, bridging the gap between resilience work and bereavement—essentially developing a new concept of resilient grieving—gave new meaning and purpose to her life. It created something demonstratively good out of something catastrophically bad, something she could share with the world. This culminated in her writing and publishing her bestselling book, *Resilient Grieving*.

As a part of resilient grieving, Dr. Hone encourages people to allow themselves to feel *all* the feelings—not just those we've been conditioned to view as reasonable. This means that we must check our judgment when we're feeling angry or fearful, hurt, or numb and allow ourselves to feel and express these, too. Just as importantly, when we're "supposed" to be grieving, we must resist punishing ourselves for moments of joy or humor or silliness that we might get swept up in. When we accept all our feelings, we step more fully into our humanness and become more fully available to experience whatever life throws our way. I saw this firsthand in a young patient of mine, Miriam.

Miriam was only twenty-seven when she came to me after suffering a few bouts of severe shortness of breath coupled with severe heart palpitations. She told me she felt as if she might be having a heart attack. I gave her a complete workup, and fortunately nothing suggested any heart problems. But that didn't mean something wasn't terribly wrong: I could tell, when she began to describe her symptoms, how real and debilitating they were.

A year earlier, she'd been promoted at the consulting firm where she worked, which meant she would have to travel quite a bit. I asked her if she enjoyed this. "Yes. Or at least usually I do. But during this last trip, to London, I started experiencing this chest pain and dizziness and shortness of breath."

I asked her if she had been under any undue stress while on the job, or if anything had changed in her life recently. "Well"—she hesitated—"my father passed away, unexpectedly, two weeks before this last work trip, so I only had time to go home to Michigan for the funeral. I knew I didn't feel up to going on this trip, but I didn't feel comfortable asking my boss for more time off."

I could feel my eyes welling up as she spoke. She told me that it wasn't that her boss wasn't understanding; in fact, her boss had offered her more time off. But Miriam, who was new to this kind of loss and this level of grief, felt that she ought to be "okay" and carry on and act as though she hadn't just lost her beloved father. She told me she'd been numb when she said goodbye to her mother and numb when she boarded the plane for England. But as soon as she landed, she'd begun having these terrifying symptoms. "I just muscled my way through those four days, landed back in New York City, and went to the ER. That's when I was referred to you."

When she finished this story, I could see every muscle in her body relax. Now I understood. Miriam had felt compelled to hide her feelings of grief and vulnerability from her boss and coworkers, and this incredible suppression of her emotions had brought on what I realized were a series of panic attacks.

Panic attacks occur when we're under so much stress that it triggers a hormonal response, activating our fight, flight, or freeze response, which then leads to an overwhelming adrenaline rush, as I described in the previous chapter. This causes us to experience some of the same symptoms we may see in people experiencing arrhythmia (irregular heartbeat), which can feel like palpitations, or a racing or irregular heartbeat. Other patients experience symptoms such as chest pain, shortness of breath, sweating, and tingling or numbness in their hands. I sent Miriam for a full workup to rule out an arrhythmia or some other heart condition. Fortunately, her tests came back negative. Once we recognized that what Miriam was experiencing were likely panic attacks, we were able to focus on the why.

Panic attacks, although terrifying and often debilitating when happening, are usually short-lived (subsiding within minutes) and are not fatal. Miriam had many unexpressed feelings related to her father's untimely death, leaving her mother on her own, and the stressors of her demanding new position at work. What she needed most was *not* to act as if everything were okay and to hustle across the Atlantic to the next big client meeting, but rather the time, space, and support to unpack her feelings and come to terms with her traumatic loss. I recommended that she see a therapist to help her work through her grief, which, I suspected, was contributing to her panic attacks.

Two weeks later, she called from Michigan to say that her company had given her six weeks of paid bereavement leave and that she was now back home with her mother. She had reached out to a grief counselor there, in her hometown, who was helping both her and her mother come to terms with their loss. Six weeks later, when she came back into my office, she reported that she felt refreshed and that the time she'd been able to spend with her mother was incredibly healing—for both of them. She felt confident that she and her mother, whom she had grown even closer to, would stay in close touch and continue to work through and process their grief together. She was also continuing her own therapy with a counselor in New York who had come highly recommended to her by a work colleague. Miriam, I learned, was beginning to open up; she no longer felt compelled to bury her feelings and act as though her father's death had not affected her. Most important, she had not had a panic attack since our initial visit. I was happy to send her off, after a big warm hug, knowing that her heart health was intact, and that she was working on processing her feelings—which involved, in no small part, grieving for her father and therefore building her resilience.

Some of us, like Miriam, believe these feelings should have some kind of time limit. But what Dr. Hone began to understand in her research, which she shared with me, is that grief is a new facet of our lives that will be with us forever.

Trying to bury grief doesn't serve us—or our memory of those closest to us. When someone dies, our love for them does not. We emerge changed by the experience both of having had them in our lives, and by the experience of losing them.

One of the transformative practices Dr. Hone created for herself simply requires taking out a pen and a piece of paper and asking and answering these questions:

- What did the person you lost teach you?
- How did he or she change you?
- How will you live in and relate differently to the world because they were in it?

What this practice does is transform the best of the person we lost (their zest for life, their thoughtfulness, their sense of humor) into a powerful positive touchstone that we can then carry forward with us, allow-

Accept Your Current Situation

ing them to continue to enrich our lives even as we walk on through life without them by our side. This simple act of remembrance allows us to carry our loved one's essence forward into the here and now. It's a way to accept a new reality, without burying your grief.

Dr. Hone was thinking of Abi's bubbly, joyful spirit when she saw Abi's stark-white coffin. So Dr. Hone reached out to an artistic friend and asked for her help in decorating the casket so that it would reflect Abi's personality. Her friend had multicolored plastic dots made and asked Dr. Hone, her husband, and their sons to affix them to the coffin. Everyone who came to pay their respects added another. By the time of Abi's burial, her coffin was covered in brightly colored dots. (When Dr. Hone told me this story, she mentioned that all these years later, she still has a colored dot attached to the back of her phone.) People wore the dots on their lapels or put them on their cars. The colored dots were disbursed to all of Abi's friends, and even now, a decade after her death, Dr. Hone will get pictures of an Abi Dot on the Louvre in Paris, or the Brooklyn Bridge—Abi's now-young-adult friends keep her spirit alive by continuing to place her dots at beautiful places all over the world.

Dr. Hone also wears a lovely brooch, which she bought when she was with Abi, whenever she speaks, and she told me that she felt as though Abi had, in very real and profound ways, written her book with her, knowing that she would never have explored and discovered resilient grieving without losing her daughter.

For Miriam, keeping her father close meant putting her favorite photograph of her with her parents on her desk at work, their arms around one another, the three of them laughing uncontrollably. Creating a living legacy such as this is a gorgeous way to keep a loved one's spirit alive within us. I cannot think of a better way to illustrate the healing power of a resilient spirit than this. Because a key part of a living legacy is that word *living*—which those of us left behind must continue to do.

Sometimes, though, there is no single incident we can point to as the cause of our grief. This happens when we suffer from ambiguous loss, which lacks the clarity and certainty that comes when there is a clear event, such as a death. This ambiguity can complicate and prolong grieving.

Examples of ambiguous loss include someone's physical absence even when they might be present in your mind and thoughts, as in cases of disappearance, abandonment, deportation, divorce, or separation. A second type of ambiguous loss is the reverse: psychological absence despite physical presence. This can occur with mental illnesses, such as severe depression or psychosis; with workaholism, addictions, or affairs; or as the result of cognitive decline, as in Alzheimer's, where the person is physically present but altered or emotionally unavailable.

Ambiguous loss can have a profound impact on both our physical and mental well-being. The prolonged stress brought on by this ongoing uncertainty can manifest in the same physical symptoms as other types of chronic stress, including a weakened immune system, cardiovascular problems, and sleep disturbances, and in mental health conditions such as anxiety and depression. Our relationships with others in our life may suffer, and even daily functioning might become difficult as we question our place in the world. Recognizing ambiguous loss and seeking support through therapy, support groups, or specialized resources is crucial for those of us navigating this complex grief experience. Loss of anything—an important person in our life, a relationship, a long-held goal, a job that helped us

Accept Your Current Situation

form an identity—can lead us to grieve, so when we get a new diagnosis or are confronted with a change in our medical status, learning to accept it can be critical. A medical diagnosis or a loss—or both, like we've seen in this chapter—requires that we accept a change of goalposts, as Dr. Hone explained. But it doesn't mean we can't make thoughtful, considered, and aligned new goals.

It all goes back to the practice of accepting what we cannot change and *learning to change* what we can—that is where a flexible mindset comes in, which we will explore next.

CHAPTER 4

Embrace Flexible Thinking

When BJ Miller was a nineteen-year-old sophomore at Princeton University, he and his friends who'd been out for drinks decided, at 4:00 a.m., that it would be fun to climb a parked commuter railcar. BJ went first. He scampered up the ladder on the back of the car, and once he was out of sight, his friends heard an explosion and saw a big flash of light. BJ was wearing a metal watch, which acted as a conduit for the live electrical wires strung above the train car. As he stepped onto its roof, he was hit with eleven thousand volts of electricity, which coursed down his left arm and through his legs. The power of the electrical shock threw him off his feet. He landed on the roof of the car. Without hesitation, his friend Pete scrambled up and found BJ bleeding from the head, his body *smoking*. While Pete worked to keep BJ calm, his friend Jonathan was on the ground calling 911. BJ stayed conscious while police and ambulance workers worked a stretcher up onto the train-car roof—at great danger to all of them—and strapped BJ in and got him down and to the ER. He was in excruciating pain, as the electrical current had burned him from the inside out, speeding through his body and exiting through the tips of his fingers and toes.

The Healing Power of Resilience

When Miller awoke several days later in the burn unit at St. Barnabas Medical Center in New Jersey, he felt as if he were coming out of a bad dream. Unaware of his condition, he pulled off IV lines and unhooked himself from monitors and tried to hobble to the bathroom, until he wrenched the catheter from his body and fell to the floor in excruciating pain. He spent the next month in the burn unit, in a touch-and-go state, living, as he's described it, in a place that toggled between life and death. Then things stabilized some and he was there for another month, then another, and another; all totaled, he was in the burn unit for four months, often in isolation, as there is such a high risk of infection for those with serious burns. Doctors first amputated both of his legs just below the knee. But then it came time to take his arm, and this struck Miller hard. He remembers the hallway between his room and the elevator that would take him down to the operating room was lined with his family and friends. He felt, he has said, both seen and loved, and this reassured him that he would make it through what was for him an unimaginable loss.

He came out of surgery, and the first person he saw was his mother, who had always inspired him but now did more than ever. His mother had polio when she was a child, and as often happens with polio survivors, she experienced postpolio syndrome as a young adult. Miller remembers, as a child, his mother with braces on her legs or using crutches and still being physically active. But when she was in her forties, her condition began to progressively degenerate, culminating with her needing to use an electric wheelchair. He understood, by his mother's example, that this kind of physical change was *just part of life*. She modeled for him how to accept and continue to live a full, rich, and meaningful life, without allowing her disability to define her. Because of her example, and his new awareness that the body is fragile and temporary, Miller never allowed himself to wallow in the "Why me?" of self-pity and despair for too long, though he's honest that these feelings arose, for sure. Miller had always been sensitive to suffering and loss, but now he embraced that truth in a way that allowed him to dwell in an incredibly attuned space—the space where all of us will one day experience suffering and loss not as a disruption, but as an inevitable part of this fragile thing we call life. He made a conscious choice to see himself as a vital part of the world around him, now in a different body from the one he had before. This allowed him to expand his perspective on what it meant to be lovable, able, and, most important, meaningfully connected to others.

After a year, he returned to Princeton a changed man. He was no longer the six-foot-five athlete with the movie-star good looks; he was the guy with the prosthetic limbs and a service dog and got around campus in a golf cart. He originally planned to major in Chinese and do some kind of humanitarian work abroad, but he switched his major to art history, wanting to immerse himself in exploring how we humans create art as a way of making sense of the world. As he said to Krista Tippett in a 2016 interview, "This radical change to my body offered this great excuse to refashion my perspective, refashion and 'compose' my sense of self." But this, he is careful to point out, wasn't easy to do; he had tremendous pain, both physical and psychological, to work through. He began to reimagine what a meaningful, productive life might look like, and how he might be different as a person, too.

He graduated from Princeton, then worked in arts advocacy and disability rights for a while, but then medicine began to call to him. While he was finishing medical school, his older sister and only sibling died by suicide. At the time of her death, Miller was becoming disillusioned with the prospect of pursuing a career as a doctor—until he stumbled upon a palliative-care course while he was an intern at the Medical College of Wisconsin. This was the game changer for Miller.

Palliative care is a relatively new specialty in medicine, and its successful practice has much to do with both step one and two of the Resilience Response: acceptance and flexibility of mindset. In 1990, the World Health Organization (WHO) recognized it as a distinct specialty concerned with relieving the suffering and improving the quality of life for people who had suffered grievous injury or were facing a debilitating, chronic, or life-threatening illness. Not until 2006 did the American Board of Medical Specialties recognize it in the United States. Because palliative care is all about nurturing a patient—whereas most of medicine is concerned with identifying the problem (diagnosis) and solving it (finding a cure), it is often grouped with hospice care. But there is an important distinction between the two. Whereas hospice care is focused on alleviating suffering and pain at the end of life, palliative care focuses on the holistic well-being of a patient who is actively pursuing treatment or a cure for a serious disease or illness, with the hope that there is still potential for recovery—and this is something Miller had personal experience with. Palliative care is all about restoring and maintaining quality of life—and it was that aspect of the specialty that spoke to him. At its core, the specialty's aim is to reduce suffering by offering multidisciplinary support (pain management, symptom management, psychological and spiritual support) that ensures that a patient's sense of self is not lost during treatment, that his or her illness does not become their identity.

People who face serious, even life-threatening, illnesses, including heart diseases such as congestive heart failure (CHF), benefit from palliative care. With the support of a palliative care team (which I think of as the "quality of life" team), patients demonstrably live longer and report a higher quality of life, despite often facing a daunting prognosis. A meta-analysis conducted by the National Institutes of Health on the impact of palliative care looked at quality of life as connected to how the patient perceived fulfillment of personal goals, control of physical symptoms, emotional well-being, the ability to maintain a sense of self, the ability to maintain one's role within family and society, finding fulfillment and meaning in life, and recalibration of goals in light of disease trajectory. The analysis of multiple systematic reviews and randomized controlled trials found palliative care interventions do improve quality of life among patients with advanced diseases.

BJ Miller explained that coming to grips with his injuries and the severe pain from them was a long process—and one that he was only able to get through due to the support of so many around him, including the kind and compassionate medical professionals who treated him. They understood that easing back into life was a process, and that it would entail learning to live with loss, pain, and sorrow. What these people did was listen, stand by him, and constantly validate his experience, however hard it was. This is what palliative care is all about.

When I had the chance to sit down with Miller, now a hospice and palliative care doctor on the faculty of the University of California, San Francisco School of Medicine, he talked about how learning to accept loss, pain, and sorrow as essential parts of life is vital. It allowed him to change his perspective. He realized that we are all in this dance with life and death, and that grounded him. It is also, as he's quick to point out, what put him more profoundly in touch with beauty, joy, and love. It also showed him that, if he could survive and recover from something such as being electrocuted, he could learn how to live in his forever-changed body and find new meaning in what was now possible for him, which was a different version of what was possible in the body he was born into. He had to change how he was thinking about his future. And that's why, after acceptance, learning to adopt a flexible mindset is the next step of the Resilience Response.

Unlike BJ Miller, I always knew I wanted to be a doctor—I didn't need a catastrophe to tell me that. But my path to actually becoming one was a little less than straight—it similarly required transformation, a major deviation from my original planned career path, which wouldn't have been possible if I hadn't expanded my thinking.

I grew up in Florida. When I was just a child, my father would take me on rounds with him at the hospital. One of the things I remember so profoundly was that my father would always lay a hand on a patient, patting the leg of a bedridden patient or placing a gentle touch on a shoulder or forehead. I loved that. I was the kid who always rushed over to a friend or classmate whenever they skinned a knee and offered to clean and bandage them. And I loved everything science related, even going to science camp in the summers. So when I went off to get my undergraduate degree at Stanford University, I went thinking I'd major in premed, but my father, surprisingly, was very discouraging about my going into medicine. He knew how grueling the hours were and that it would be especially hard for me, as a woman, if I wanted to also have a family. He thought there were other ways I could make money, so he advocated for me to major in business. I love my father, and I appreciated his frankness, so I took his advice and majored in economics with a minor in biology.

I did well at Stanford, but I never really clicked with my fellow business majors, who couldn't wait to graduate and join a well-heeled Wall Street firm or some hot Silicon Valley venture-capital group. I had no desire to do either of these things, so what on earth would I do with a business degree? With no clear path forward, I flew home

Embrace Flexible Thinking

to Florida to live with my parents and figure it out. I did know that I wanted to work for myself, and I wanted to do something creative, but what? First I thought about opening a restaurant—maybe I could do that back in California? My parents gently tried to convey to me how tough the restaurant business is and how it might be hard for me, a new college graduate who was all of twenty-one, to open a restaurant across the country. I realized they had a point. Maybe, then, I could open a restaurant in Miami? At least then I could live at home while I figured out how to get it off the ground. This, my parents felt, was also not the wisest of plans. So I scaled back my thinking and decided to open a smoothie shop. Jamba Juice was just taking off in California—why not create something similar here? So, three months out of college, I flew back to California to figure out how Jamba Juice worked.

I would never have predicted that in my first job out of Stanford I would be wearing an orange visor and whipping up smoothies for undergrads eight hours a day, but that's exactly what I did. Every night, I'd go home to my budget-hotel room and write down everything I'd learned that day: from how many crates of oranges to order, to how to clean and fix an overused blender, to what a payroll was. After a couple of months, with a full notebook and a pretty good sense of what it took to run a juice bar, I flew back to Miami.

Then I bought a book on how to write a business plan. I studied that book, wrote a plan, then shared it with my parents, who then graciously offered to help me with the start-up costs for Sun Juice, my soon-to-be smoothie bar. I cannot overstate how crucial my parents' belief in me was to making this vision a reality.

Next, I signed the lease on a great little retail space in Coral Gables, created a logo featuring an Egyptian goddess, and wrote a mythical origin story about Sun Juice that I hung on the wall.

The Healing Power of Resilience

It took me nine months to get Sun Juice off the ground, but at just twenty-two years old, I had twelve to fifteen employees and a successful business. I was written up as a hot young entrepreneur in *New Times* magazine, and we were rated the number one smoothie bar in town. I had done it. And it was incredibly gratifying and satisfying. But once I'd done the hard work of creating the business and proving to myself and the world at large that it was sustainable and profitable, my creative juices began pulling me in another direction. Launching Sun Juice was terrifying, grueling, thrilling, and ultimately successful. But at the end of the day, I just wasn't happy. Even though my business was successful, I was miserable.

One night, while we were sitting around the dinner table, I finally blurted out, "I can't do this anymore!"

My mother said, "Do what anymore?"

I had no choice but to tell my parents I couldn't run Sun Juice anymore. When they asked me why not, I told them that making money and helping people in this limited way wasn't fulfilling enough, that I needed to contribute to society beyond frozen drinks. This was the moment of truth: Despite my crying now, I told them I wanted to become a doctor, that being a physician, I knew, was my true calling. I had gone a long way down the road of becoming an entrepreneur, but it wasn't the path I wanted to continue on. I needed to accept the "sunk costs" in time and effort and money and move on in a new direction.

That night was a turning point for me, and I knew I would never have gotten there if I hadn't first opened and run my own business. My parents, to their credit, couldn't have been more supportive. I had to enroll in additional undergraduate classes to finish the premed requirements I had started at Stanford. I also studied for and took the MCAT (and the GMAT, just in case), then sent out applications to medical schools and held my breath. Was opening myself to new experiences, to the potential for failure, to the unknown, going to work out?

I got into George Washington University's medical school and was excited about the prospect of studying in Washington, DC. But then, seemingly at the last minute, I got a letter from the Keck School of Medicine at the University of Southern California. I got in! And so, at age twenty-four, I went back to the West Coast to pursue the next part of my education.

But I didn't abandon Sun Juice; instead, I left the management of the company in the very capable hands of my parents, who ran it and then successfully sold it in 2001. I'm proud to say that Sun Juice is still open today, in the exact same location, and when I go home to visit, I get to bring my kids there.

My story and BJ Miller's story don't have altogether that much in common, but one thing we shared was maintaining a flexible mindset in the face of the unexpected, a willingness to switch course to accommodate change. BJ's life was, after all, remade in an instant.

Have you ever heard the expression "Be the river, not the rock"? I've always taken this to mean to try to "go with flow," to let life happen—rather than stubbornly clinging to what we think life ought to be. A longtime patient of mine taught me a lesson about how important flexibility can be. Claudia is an actively practicing psychologist in her seventies who initially came to me for her blood pressure and risk-factor management. Over the years she had had a few possible TIAs (transient ischemic attacks, or ministrokes). When she came to me after the first one, she was terrified—the symptoms had shown up out of nowhere as an abrupt change in her speech and thoughts while she was talking on the phone. Afterward she had issues with word searching and what she felt was a lag between thought and speech. Though her full workup yielded no evidence of a stroke, that it was likely a TIA meant we had to look at whether a clot from inside or outside the heart had temporarily blocked oxygenated blood from reaching the brain. She had all kinds of tests and assessments, but the cause of the TIA was not determined.

And so Claudia lived in fear every day. It was as if her whole world had been turned upside down, and she had no idea if or when it might happen again or what the next result would be. We spoke about how this was normal, and how allowing some time to pass might give her some clarity and perspective and a feeling of more safety. As each day passed and she was able to continue her life and practice with no further events, she grew more confident and peaceful. She regained her footing, and not until just this past year has she again had an episode that seemed consistent with another ministroke. This time, however, she was not rocked by the event but seemed calm as she relayed to me what had happened. She told me she remembered our initial conversation and how helpful it had been. She also said how lucky she felt to have found me when she did on her health journey, which made me feel grateful. She also asked me if I had ever heard the story of the Zen farmer. I hadn't, and she emailed me a link to the story.

The parable is of a farmer who faces many challenges. He learns that what at first might seem like a bad event ends up being a good event in his life. He learns you can't always tell at first when something happens whether the outcome will be bad or good. His response becomes "Bad luck. Good luck. Who knows?" I loved this story so much I shared it with my entire family—and took from it the idea that our perspective needs to remain open, our mind needs to stay flexible. Life can and will throw obstacles in our way, and if we can retain equanimity, we can ride the wave until we see if it has brought us somewhere good or bad.

Every one of us will face failure, loss, and uncertainty in our lives. That's why a flexible mindset is such an important aspect of resilience.

When we face any health issue, or any stressor, with an open mind, we can overcome incredible challenges.

Steven Hayes, whom we met in the previous chapter, wrote about how to do that. He coined the term *psychological flexibility* back in the mid-1980s and has, helpfully, spent the subsequent forty years thinking about what that looks like in practice.

Practicing psychological flexibility, he says, is broken down into three pillars. The first is awareness. When something happens, take the time to notice, to observe. Watch passively as thoughts, feelings, and sensations bubble up. This exercise flows naturally into the next pillar, openness. Once we have a sense of what emotions we are experiencing, our job is to accept them, no matter how painful or negative they may be. As Hayes puts it, this step is all about "dropping the internal fight," which then, perhaps counterintuitively, allows feelings to *become* more positive overall. Finally, the third pillar is valued engagement. This, the most active step, asks us to take the time to assess our goals. Now that we know how we're feeling and we aren't fighting the bad stuff anymore, it's our job to figure out what really matters and where we want to go.

Easy enough, right?

While Hayes provides a framework for attaining this flexible mindset, it's not always as simple as it may seem. Sometimes, we need a little push to show us that we can engage with a challenge or a hardship in this way.

The Power of Denial

You may think that denial can be harmful when encountering a challenge. I just spent the previous chapter talking about the importance of acceptance!

But let me tell you about Richard Cohen.

The Healing Power of Resilience

When I was struggling with my eyesight, I read a book called *Blindsided: Lifting a Life Above Illness*, by Richard Cohen. Cohen, who called the book a "reluctant memoir," was diagnosed with MS at twenty-five, survived two bouts of colon cancer, was legally blind for much of his life, and yet had an incredible, award-winning career as a war correspondent and journalist. He was married to journalist Meredith Viera for almost forty years and was the father of three children. Sadly, he passed away in late 2024 after a struggle with pneumonia.

I had the chance to speak with Richard twenty years after I first read his book. He was a third-generation MS patient: Both his grandmother and his father had MS. What he learned by their example, especially his father, was not to allow himself to be victimized by the illness—to accept it and live with it rather than in spite of it. Indeed, his father, a physician, practiced medicine for nearly four decades and lived into his nineties. He taught Richard, by example, that he could live a rich and meaningful life while having MS. Richard had seen others close to him do it, and he told himself that meant so could he. Though the diagnosis was devastating, maintaining a flexible mindset helped him see that he could nonetheless continue to pursue his dreams—living with, not despite, his illness.

That's a little bit different of a tactic from Miller's, who reimagined his life after his accident. Richard just . . . kept going. Neither fought the bad stuff; they just went where they wanted to go.

Richard was not in any position to stop or give up. When he learned he had MS, he was only twenty-five and had just landed a plumb position as a producer with ABC News. A neurologist he had only seen once called and blurted out that Richard had MS, and that there was no treatment and no cure. And then hung up. "Diagnosed and adios. Nothing much we can do," Richard recalled. "I remember thinking, 'Wow. This sucks. But I don't have enough information about this to freak out, so I won't.' And I didn't. But I also didn't talk about it. There was, and remains, way too much stigma put on people who have to go through life with a chronic illness, so I decided that I would just go ahead and live my life."

I asked Richard if he thought of this as stoicism, and he laughed. "I'd actually use the word *denial*. Look—I wasn't in denial about having MS. What I mean by denial is I wasn't about to let this disease dictate the terms of my life, you know? I wasn't going to let it keep me from getting the jobs I wanted, which eventually included reporting from war zones and having to run my ass off so I wouldn't get shot."

Cohen certainly piqued my interest in adding the concept of denial to my understanding of resilience. It was completely at odds with the pillars of Hayes's definition, and yet, Cohen arrived at a similar destination: He knew what really mattered to him.

"Of course, I told the people I'm close to about my illness. I told Meredith, my wife, on our second date because I wanted her to know what she might be getting herself into. But she decided she was interested in me anyway, and we've been together ever since." Richard had a strong marriage and a close bond with his children—which are absolutely relationship goals for me.

But he wasn't an open book, either. "Aside from only those closest to me knowing, my father encouraged me, from early on, not to share my illness with anyone else. He knew the stigma that would get attached to me, and he wanted me to define my life on my own terms and not become my diagnosis." And so, in a sense, his keeping this private became a kind of denial, too—he only shared his full self with a chosen few, but with the rest of the world, he refused to accept their preconceived notions that would come along with their knowledge of his MS.

The Healing Power of Resilience

Cohen didn't make his diagnosis public until deep into his career, when he was a well-established producer for the *Evening News with Walter Cronkite*. Only after he'd proven himself on the job did he share with his bosses that he had MS. "I wanted them to already know how capable I was; I didn't want someone else to decide what I could or couldn't do."

As a point of illustration, when he was interviewed by Barbara Walters on the publication of *Blindsided* in 2004, Walters asked him, incredulously, why he still took the subway. "Because I can" was his answer.

My conversation with Cohen opened up a whole new way of thinking about denial for me. I asked him to elaborate on this, and he said, "If you're standing on a train track and there's a train coming toward you and you deny it's going to hit you, then you're making a big mistake. But if denial means denying the certainty of possible future outcomes, that's a totally different story. And that kind of denial, for me, is a formula for living. For going on with my life."

I was beginning to understand; if being in denial meant not letting anyone else dictate how well or how long he'd function while having MS, I could get on board with that. Cohen consciously shied away from listening to others, who, he told me, often want to make us feel that we're victims—even when we don't see ourselves that way.

"Look. It's not like I don't get frustrated. Or angry or have a down day. But I believe now, and I've always believed, that to see yourself as the victim is a terrible mistake. You've just got to play the cards you've been dealt, and you've just got to keep going."

Richard Cohen used what he called denial to keep limitation settings at bay. He met life's challenges head-on and course-corrected as needed to continue to fulfill his purpose of doing tough, meaningful work, being a great role model for his children, and walking through life, with humor and devotion, beside his wife.

I asked him if he had any final thoughts on resilience and he shared this: "I believe people are stronger than they think they are. They sell themselves short. But most of us don't find out how strong we are until we're tested. And when you're tested, if you don't psych yourself out or let other people psych you out, you'll find out just how strong you are." When he passed away, I felt a deep sadness for the man whose ideas and life had helped me so much at a time when I was struggling desperately to find my way through my own health challenge.

The Power of Believing

Cohen's thinking got me, in turn, thinking about other mindset shifts that might be helpful as you practice the Resilience Response.

There is a well-documented but still somewhat mysterious phenomenon in medicine known as the placebo effect. This occurs when a patient shows objective improvement, such as a lessening of symptoms, when the only treatment they receive is the *suggestion* that they're being given some kind of medical intervention that will make them better, rather than their actually being treated with any kind of drug or intervention. For instance, being given a pill that they are told contains medication, but is actually just inert sugar or another harmless substance.

Placebo is derived from the Latin phrase for "I shall please," and the placebo effect has been observed since ancient times, and even back then, it took on the cast of being some kind of sham or medical parlor trick. This was in the era of bleeding, blistering, purging, and all kinds of other medical quackery and pseudoscience. But beginning in the eighteenth century, the placebo effect as an actual prompt for healing began to be recognized, and in the nineteenth century, with the advent of modern, empirically based medicine, it was acknowledged as such.

It was still mistrusted because it couldn't be quantified or specifically identified. But with the twentieth-century shift to a medical culture built firmly on the use of clinical trials to test the efficacy of drugs and other treatments, the placebo effect became a standard variable and finally found itself gaining legitimacy when used as the control factor in clinical drug trials. This is when our understanding of the vast power of the placebo effect finally began to kick in. A key figure in this shift was Henry K. Beecher, a Harvard anesthesiologist. In the 1950s, Beecher's research highlighted the powerful influence of the mind on the body. He demonstrated that placebos could produce significant effects on pain, anxiety, and other symptoms, even in controlled clinical trials. Beecher found that in fifteen trials with different diseases, 35 percent of patients were satisfactorily relieved by a placebo alone, an oft-cited statistic.

We've known about the placebo effect for centuries but we're only beginning to understand how it triggers actual healing. When we're told something will make us feel better or may even cure us, we transform that suggestion into a belief. And if we hold that belief, we have the potential to initiate an actual neurobiological response in which neurotransmitters trigger the release of hormones, and our immune response is heightened. When this happens, not only do we experience a sense of well-being and a resulting reduction in our levels of stress, but we may also experience a lessening of symptoms such as pain or inflammation or anxiety. In one remarkable study on knee surgery for osteoarthritis, patients underwent either actual arthroscopic surgery for the condition, or a sham surgery where incisions were made but no actual surgical procedure was performed inside the knee. Incredibly, the two groups reported similar levels of pain relief and improved function, despite that no intervention had actually occurred in the placebo group.

Embrace Flexible Thinking

Two primary theories have been proposed to explain the placebo effect. One, the mentalistic theory, posits that the placebo effect is driven by a patient's beliefs and expectations. When a patient believes a treatment will be effective, their brain releases neurotransmitters that can alleviate pain and reduce anxiety. The other theory, the Pavlovian theory, suggests that the placebo effect is a learned response, similar to classical conditioning—as when Pavlov rang a bell while giving a dog a treat, and thereafter the dog would salivate when the bell was rung even if no treat was given. It works in humans, too: If we associate past positive experiences with treatments, even if they were placebos, we can condition the body to respond positively to future placebos. For example, if someone received a medication that effectively alleviated pain in the past, subsequent placebos may trigger a similar response, even without the active ingredient.

Whatever the reasons for the power of the placebo effect, it certainly doesn't mean that we can simply "believe" our way to being cured of serious illnesses or diseases. In fact, the idea that we can somehow "will" ourselves to overcome things such as cancer or heart disease is dangerous. Willpower, or a willingness to "fight," is never enough when medical intervention is necessary to eradicate or slow the progression of a serious illness or disease. But what the placebo effect does show us is that, if we're encouraged to believe that we can get better, our brain responds in a way that changes how our body responds.

Alia Crum, the American psychologist and the director of the Mind & Body Lab at Stanford University, is renowned for her research on the placebo effect and how it demonstrably influences health outcomes. Her work includes studying how social and psychological forces influence outcomes for patients with chronic diseases.

Crum first became intrigued by the placebo affect when she was still an undergraduate studying psychology at Harvard. She played on the women's ice hockey team and prided herself on always going the extra mile, spending additional time in the gym beyond regular team workouts. One day her academic adviser, psychology professor Ellen Langer, offhandedly said, "You know exercise is just a placebo, right?" This stopped Crum in her tracks and made her think: Was she in great shape because she was spending so much time in the gym, or was she fit because she *believed* that spending time in the gym was making her so?

This prompted Crum to write the mission statement she still pursues today: "To help improve people's health and happiness through increased understanding of the mind-body connection."

She conducted one of her first formal studies specifically to see how mindset might affect the efficacy of exercise. Under Langer's guidance, Crum enlisted eighty-four female housekeepers from a variety of local hotels to participate in her study. She asked all of them if they exercised regularly. Most said no, and a third said they never exercised at all. Then Crum told half of the group that their work—dusting, vacuuming, changing beds—was a meaningful form of exercise, and that they were likely meeting the recommended daily minimum standards set by the US surgeon general to promote overall health.

One month later, Crum checked in with all the study participants and discovered something astounding: The group of women who now thought of their work as a form of exercise had lost weight and lowered their blood pressure, even though they had made no changes to their lifestyle. The control group, which had not been told that their work was a form of exercise, showed no changes in their health status. Crum and Langer published their findings in the journal *Psychological Science* in 2007 and wrote that the "results support the hypothesis that exercise affects health in part or in whole via the placebo effect."

Another remarkable experiment that shows the power of the placebo effect has been immortalized as "the milkshake" experiment. In it, Crum and her colleagues at the Yale Center for Clinical and Translational Research wanted to see how our beliefs might affect us physiologically, and in particular how those beliefs might affect the activity of ghrelin, a hormone produced in the gastrointestinal system that signals hunger. In simple terms, the more ghrelin your body produces, the hungrier you will feel. The design of the study was ingenious: A set of subjects would drink two vastly different milkshakes, first one, then the other a week later. After consuming each shake, the participants' blood would be drawn and the researchers would look at the ghrelin response to each shake. The test subjects were told that one shake they'd have was a delicious confection loaded with sugar and fat and contained 620 calories. The other shake, they were told, was a low-fat, low-sugar "diet" shake that had only 140 calories. In reality the shakes were the same and contained moderate amounts of fat and sugar and had 380 calories. Crum and her team expected the diet shake to have a more positive effect on their subjects' metabolism, but the results proved otherwise: After consuming the "indulgent" shake, the subjects' ghrelin levels dropped. After drinking the "diet" shake, their ghrelin levels remained steady or even increased. The difference in ghrelin production and levels was significant, at roughly a factor of three.

What this experiment demonstrated, perhaps for the first time, is that what one believes about what one is consuming has a demonstrable metabolic effect on the body. When subjects were told they were consuming an indulgent shake, one that would be highly satiating, their brain—and their body—got the message that their hunger would be satisfied. And so it was. Not only did these subjects feel more "full," but ghrelin production slowed and the metabolic mechanisms that respond to incoming nutrition kicked into gear. On consuming what they were told was a diet shake, the subjects' brains and bodies got the obverse message: This drink will be good for me but it will not be satisfying. This messaging prompted their bodies to keep their ghrelin levels steady or to actually increase their ghrelin levels, as the message received was "This food is not satisfying." Additionally, the metabolic systems that process nutrition stayed quiet.

The difference in the ghrelin response was striking and definitively proved that *what we believe* about what we're eating affects how our bodies respond physiologically to that food. What fascinated Crum was how counterintuitive the study results were. As Crum put it on an episode of the *Huberman Lab* podcast, "When these participants thought they were eating sensibly, their bodies still left them feeling physiologically hungry, while those who believed they were eating indulgently, their bodies responded that they had had enough food." This indicates that a mindset of deprivation may not be the best mindset for controlling ghrelin production and might therefore not be the best mindset for positively influencing the body's metabolic function around diet and weight loss.

These early studies launched Crum's ongoing, groundbreaking work, which continues to broaden our understanding of how mindset influences our health.

Another profound example of how our thinking can influence our health outcomes is found in what is called the nocebo effect. The nocebo effect, the opposite of the placebo effect, occurs when negative expectations lead to negative health outcomes. Derived from the Latin word *nocere*, meaning "to harm," this phenomenon again shows the powerful influence of the mind on the body.

Embrace Flexible Thinking

When patients anticipate adverse effects from a treatment, they become more susceptible to experiencing them. This heightened awareness can trigger physiological responses, such as increased heart rate, muscle tension, or changes in hormone levels. The nocebo effect can have significant implications for patient care. For instance, negative publicity or misinformation about a medication can lead to increased reporting of adverse effects, even if the drug is safe and effective. Or, when a brand-name drug is advertised as more effective or as a gold standard for treatment, patients may experience increased side effects when switching to a generic version, even if the two medications are chemically identical. Negative expectations about a medical procedure, such as surgery, can also increase anxiety and pain, potentially leading to poorer outcomes. This is a powerful reminder of how what you think can play a key role in medical outcomes.

Mindset as a Tool

Mindset is one of most exciting areas of study emerging in the worlds of psychology and neurobiology. So far in this chapter, we've seen how changing our mindset can change how individuals respond to one of life's biggest stressors—as both Miller and Cohen did—but mindset can also help with life's daily stressors, such as dealing with finances or parenting responsibilities. As we discussed earlier, chronic stress is one of the biggest enemies to health and well-being, so if our mindset can be a tool when we inevitably encounter stress, big or small, this would be a transformational breakthrough.

In a 2013 TEDGlobal talk that's been viewed by more than thirty-two million people, Kelly McGonigal, a health psychologist at Stanford, confesses that for years she'd gotten stress all wrong. She believed that "stress makes you sick. It increases the risk of everything from the common cold to cardiovascular disease." But then her mind was changed when she read the 2012 study conducted at the University of Wisconsin–Madison that looked at the effect stress had on health—but with a twist. The researchers wanted to see if they could measure whether our *perception* of stress might influence its effect on us.

Using decades of metadata, the study zoomed in on a group of about thirty thousand adults who, when asked, all agreed that they were stressed. The researchers rated the level of stress as low, medium, and high. They then looked at public records eight years later to see if there was any correlation between the intensity of the stress and the mortality of this group. Participants who reported a high level of stress *and* who reported that they believed that stress affected their health in a significant way had an increased risk of premature death of 43 percent. Interestingly, what this study also showed is that the *perception* of stress as a factor in impacting health is important: in other words, you can be under incredible stress, but if you don't believe that stress will harm your health, it decreases the effect. This study demonstrates that how you think about stress—the mindset with which you approach stress—can diffuse its power to harm. Do you have a stress-accepting or a stress-combating mindset? That can make all the difference.

The study above caused McGonigal to rethink her negative stereotyping of stress and to entertain the possibility that stress may be beneficial in important ways—we've long known this about physical health, but it can also be true for mental health. McGonigal was discovering what pioneering psychologists such as Carol Dweck had been exploring about the power of a stress-accepting mindset to promote well-being. This growing body of work shows us, unequivocally, that if we view

Embrace Flexible Thinking

life's daily stressors as normal, healthy challenges and opportunities for personal growth, it changes our physiological response to that stress. McGonigal wants people to know, when they're hit with stress and recognize it via a pounding heart or sweaty palms or the urge to take immediate action, that this is your body letting you know it is prepared to meet the challenge in front of you, to know that you are resilient.

What a powerful, mindset-changing revelation!

Which is why practicing how to shift your thoughts is the second tool in the Resilience Response.

CHAPTER 5

Get Fit

In our modern lives, most of us spend far too much time sitting, whether at the wheel of a car, behind a computer monitor or phone screen, or in front of a TV. Our sedentary lifestyles and lack of physical activity have been directly linked to many health issues, including ones that are especially concerning to me, such as the onset of cardiovascular disease. Day in and day out, I find myself reminding patients—and myself, and my family—that we need to seek out good stress, the kind produced by physical exertion and exercise. This does wonders to mitigate the bad stress, the chronic wear and tear that arises when we repeatedly flood our bodies with cortisol, and to help prevent the onset of disease and protect our hearts.

My friend Andy Merlis learned this the hard way back in early November 2012. Andy is a longtime CBS News producer, former colleague, cherished friend, and . . . now my patient. In early November 2012, he was working his usual long, stressful shifts (which included more than a few all-nighters) covering major events including Hurricane Sandy. After being out in the field during the storm, he found himself more exhausted than he'd ever been in his life. Uncharacteristically, he took a few days off, but still, he couldn't shake the crushing fatigue. He woke up several days later into this weird period of malaise with what he describes as a "searing pain right in the middle of my chest." He later told me he figured it was just a severe case of heartburn (even though he rarely had it) and "swigged" some Pepto-Bismol. This helped for only a few minutes before the pain came back. He knew something was wrong and so he walked his daughter to school and then kept walking—toward the local hospital.

Along the way, he bumped into a friend he hadn't seen in years, and the two of them stood for a few moments chatting and catching up, until the friend asked Andy where he was going. "I'm walking to the hospital. I'm having some chest pain," Andy told him. The friend, surprised by this reply, hastily waved him off, and Andy walked the remaining blocks to the hospital.

Fortunately, when you walk into an ER presenting with chest pain, you're given top priority. Still, Andy was surprised when his initial blood work indicated that he was, in fact, having a heart attack. From the ER, he was whisked up to the Cath (catheterization) Lab, where he had two stents put into his obtuse marginal artery, a branch of the left circumflex artery, which supplies blood to the heart. He was forty-six years old.

When I interviewed Andy for a CBS News segment about heart health, a decade had passed since his heart attack. I asked Andy how he would describe his overall health and his lifestyle at the time of the event. He laughingly described himself as being a "gelatinous mass" then. He was a bit overweight, and his diet wasn't great; he was also under tremendous stress both on the job and at home, where he had three young kids, one with special needs. He told me he rarely gave his health much thought until that 2012 wake-up call. After that, Andy got serious about taking better care of his body. He worked on improving his diet, lost weight, and became a regular at the gym. Most important, he began to look at the stress in his life and how he could mitigate it—and change his reaction to it. He got resilient, and for Andy, as it does for many, that meant making lifestyle changes that would allow him to become healthier. He accepted his situation, thought about his life differently, and decided to get fit.

But even then, he still wasn't out of the woods. Life—including additional health issues—still came at him. In the summer of 2020, during a routine visit with me, he told me that he'd just recently run a race and was planning his next. But he also said he was having a little bit of discomfort in his chest, so I suggested another visit to the Cath Lab. That's when we found several additional blockages, including one that merited the insertion of a third stent. His blood work also showed that his glucose was, as Andy saw it, "through the roof," and although he had been diagnosed with type 2 diabetes before, he was now put on medication for it. He was fifty-four, and he says that it was tough to accept that he was, healthwise, still "a hot mess," despite all the positive lifestyle changes he'd made over the years. Andy being Andy, which is warm, hilarious, and fully engaged in life, he met—and continues to meet—these evolving health challenges head-on. He stayed resilient. "I'm not like a carpe-diem, grab-the-bull-by-the-horns kind of guy. but I am committed to living in the moment. I've learned not to look backward, not to regret things, but to just learn from them as best I can." And he's still one hell of a producer, except, as he told me, "One with a different heart: I'm a lot less cynical than I used to be, and I'm openly moved now by kindness and by people who persevere."

Luckily, Andy is doing great and he's living a full, rich life, even with chronic heart disease and diabetes. I recently learned that he'd had the word *resilience* tattooed on his arm, to remind himself how far he's come and how much living he's got left to do.

The Healing Power of Resilience

Andy is a great example of what cultivating resilience looks like in the real world. He has taken to heart all of the needed ingredients I have mentioned so far in order to build a Resilience Response: acceptance of the current situation; a flexible mindset that can allow for change; dedication to physical health through lifestyle choices such as diet, exercise, and adequate rest.

But even though the human body is designed to move, to engage in the good stress of physical activity and exertion, the medical community—especially the cardiology community—didn't always understand just how important it is to recovery.

In fact, throughout the first half of the twentieth century, prolonged, strict bed rest was the treatment of choice for heart attack sufferers. The thinking was that the heart could only heal with rest. It was believed that patients could not engage in some of the basic activities of daily life without being accompanied by an aide, including going to the bathroom or climbing a flight of stairs. Patients were often not allowed to have visitors (including family) or even to read or listen to the radio. In effect, they were treated like invalids with most of their agency—and often their dignity—taken from them. (As an aside, the same experts who insisted on full bed rest also prescribed alcohol for them, citing its calming and "vasodilating" effects.) These patients were, in essence, receiving palliative care, because the rate of survival for serious heart attack sufferers when strict bed rest was the standard of care hovered around a dismal 30 percent. Unsurprisingly, many of these patients became seriously depressed during this recovery period and lost the will to live. And now that we know exercise stimulates the release of mood-enhancing hormones called endorphins, this response makes all the more sense.

Then, in the 1950s, this all-or-nothing thinking about heart health and movement began to shift. But not without the establishment's putting up quite a fight. One of the "rebel" cardiologists who pushed back against these entrenched, draconian protocols was Bernard Lown, a cardiovascular fellow at the Peter Bent Brigham Hospital in Boston. Lown, who revolutionized cardiac care and invented lifesaving devices including both a defibrillator and a cardioverter—a device that corrects irregular heart rhythms—as well as discovering that lidocaine could be used to regulate the heartbeat, was acclaimed for his humanitarian work. As a cardiologist in training, he spoke out about the "abusive" practice of keeping heart attack sufferers lying flat and immobile, usually anywhere from four to six weeks. His insistence that cardiac patients would benefit by moving and being upright was met with unbridled hostility by the cardiology establishment. But Lown was right: Getting patients up and moving, especially in the early days following a heart event, proved to be lifesaving.

Lown conducted what is now immortalized as the "Levine chair experiment" (named for Lown's mentor, Dr. Samuel Levine). Lown recalled, in an interview recorded in 2010, seeing a patient in the 1950s "involuting" with bed rest; this man was in an oxygen tent suffocating and "gurgling" for air, likely due to what Lown believed was pulmonary edema induced because the patient was in a horizontal position, causing fluid to pool in his lungs. Lown, with his mentor by his side, moved the depressed patient out of bed and into a chair. Sitting upright allowed gravity to drain the fluid from the patient's lungs. Lown and Levine monitored the patient, whose condition and mood were markedly improved by the very next day. Within days, the patient was asking to be discharged. The staff at Peter Bent Brigham were amazed by this rapid recovery and immediately began to implement the practice of sitting cardiac patients upright. Lown and Levine followed this by putting together an informal study of eighty-one heart attack patients, and the results, though anecdotal, were equally as impressive. But despite this incredible change in outcome, the cardiology establishment remained stubborn and disdainful—even though the incidence of post-myocardial-infarction death (which deaths were caused by complications, Lown realized, of keeping patients horizontal) fell markedly. Lown described why "my approach was so vastly different: I was focused on the human being." He was not only focused on "protecting" the heart after a trauma, but took a step back to consider the health and well-being of the patient as a whole. Shifting the standard-of-care model from strict and prolonged bed rest to one of being upright and mobile drastically cut the length of hospital stays and improved mortality rates considerably.

In the 1950s, the research of Paul Dudley White, a cofounder of the American Heart Association, and a consulting physician to President Eisenhower following his heart attack in 1955, began to take hold. Dudley, who had been a medical officer during World War I, was an early user and advocate of electrocardiogram-imaging technology as a diagnostic tool in the then very new specialty of cardiology. He believed that stress management and lifestyle choices, particularly diet and exercise, were powerful influences on cardiac health long before these tools for prevention became standards of care. White was, in particular, a fan of bicycling and often advocated for taking the stairs over an elevator.

In the 1960s, scientists began to study the effects of supervised exercise on cardiac rehabilitation. The work of researchers such as Dr. Herman Hellerstein at the University of Minnesota demonstrated the safety and effectiveness of exercise in patients with heart disease and helped advocates for movement and exercise-based cardiac rehabilitation after cardiac events rather than bed rest for improving patient outcomes. Of course, the movement needed to be reintroduced slowly and with oversight. In the earliest rehabilitation programs, patients were closely monitored (by electrocardiogram, the measurement of vitals such as blood pressure and blood oxygen levels, and visual observation) as they were eased back into the everyday activity of walking. During these sessions, researchers noticed that movement also improved the mental state of the patients, including helping them overcome their fear of a recurrent event.

Today, we understand much better than did our predecessors the biological reasons for why movement helps us recover. Exercise, even after medical trauma, produces neurobiological changes that effectively mitigate the negative effects of stress on both our body and our brain. Exercise acts as a regulator, helping to reestablish homeostasis and prevent the overproduction of hormones such as cortisol. Exercise is also a catalyst for neuroplasticity; it stimulates blood flow and helps with the growth of new brain cells while strengthening existing neural connections, especially in key areas such as the hippocampus and prefrontal cortex. The release of endorphins during exercise also helps to elevate our mood and regulate our emotions. It also helps regulate immune cells and hormonal changes and leads to improved insulin sensitivity (insulin resistance is linked to increased inflammation). It keeps our heart muscle strong and our cardiovascular system working optimally; it keeps our cells, organs, and muscles strong, supple, and well functioning; and it helps prevent the onset of chronic disease by reducing inflammation, keeping our metabolic systems strong, and, importantly, protecting our mental health—all the while building up our resilience to respond to future stress.

The protective benefits of aerobic exercise are undeniable for maintaining health, particularly heart health. The American Heart Association recommends we all strive to get 150 minutes of moderate "cardio" activity (walking, biking) or 75 minutes of higher-intensity cardio activity (jogging, playing basketball) a week, if possible. Aerobic exercise strengthens the heart muscle, enabling it to pump blood more efficiently. This, in turn, reduces the pressure on arteries, leading to lower blood pressure and improved blood vessel flexibility. Exercise further benefits the entire cardiovascular system by increasing cardiac efficiency, reducing arterial stiffness, lowering stress-hormone levels, and improving blood flow. This means less buildup of plaque in our arteries and fortifies our vascular system. Lowering stress levels helps reduce chronic inflammation, helps us manage our weight, helps keep our glucose levels steady—the benefits of exercise just can't be overstated.

But aerobic exercise isn't the only kind of exercise that promotes health; new research shows how beneficial strength training is, too. A study published in *Medicine & Science in Sports & Exercise* found that lifting weights less than an hour per week can reduce your risk for heart attack or stroke by as much as 40 to 70 percent. In the past few years, strength training (specifically resistance training—such as lifting weights, doing body-weight exercises such as sit-ups, push-ups, or pull-ups, and working with resistance bands) has gotten a lot of attention due to our growing understanding of how the proteins released when skeletal muscles contract are health-promoting powerhouses. Known as myokines, these molecules help muscle-cell and tissue regeneration, stabilize metabolic processes, and have anti-inflammatory and immune-boosting properties. In strength training (when we consciously contract muscles) we release these health-boosting molecules into our bloodstream, where they work their magic throughout the body.

And recently, we've begun to understand how these proteins also work their magic on the brain, too. Stanford lecturer and health psychologist Kelly McGonigal calls myokines "hope molecules" because of the positive effect they have on our mood and mindset. In effect, myokines—or the resistance training that prompts our muscles to produce them—flood the brain with a sense of well-being and work as mood boosters. This is a different effect from the "runner's high" produced when we release endorphins during cardio-oriented workouts (such as running), but it is yet another effect that shows us how exercise is essential for promoting both mind and body wellness.

Exercising, I believe, should be enjoyable. Like a lot of people, I love cardio workouts—the feeling of getting my body working, my heart pumping; it allows me to unwind and release pent-up or negative energy. My favorite way to exercise is to put a steep incline on a treadmill and walk briskly. I also enjoy resistance training, including lifting weights. I like to feel strong and in control of my body as much as I can—especially as a woman. But it doesn't matter what form of exercise you like; I always tell patients to find something they can look forward to. Exercise can be slow and meditative, such as puttering in your garden (where we do more bending, stretching, and lifting than we realize), or rigorous, such as training for and then climbing a mountain. What is most important is not the number of steps you log but how well you can incorporate movement into your daily life so that you stay limber, your metabolic systems stay sharp, and your brain and body both get the kind of physical engagement they need to function optimally. Life isn't a race (though it may often feel like one), but it is a participation sport, and knowing that exercise is a key driver of health and a way to prevent the onset of disease gives us the *why* we need to make exercise, or just good old-fashioned physical activity, a lifestyle priority. The best kind of exercise is any activity that makes you feel good.

On the one hand, we should be heartened to know that we have such profound control over the trajectory of our health. On the other, many of us feel helpless and unable to make meaningful lifestyle changes because both the external and internal forces in our lives feel, at times, insurmountable. And, yes, I'm back to talking about stress. It's unavoidable!

This entire book is built around how stress can either be a catalyst for positive change or a driver of chronic illness and disease. Again and again, I return to our urgent need to acknowledge stress as perhaps the most pressing public health issue we currently face, and this is why we need to start putting stress reduction at the center of how we live our lives.

This is where the Resilience Response becomes so essential.

No matter what our circumstances, each of us can make even the most modest of changes to our lifestyle, particularly in the key areas of diet, exercise, and sleep. And we need to know that even small changes, taken consistently over time, will have a positive impact and will move us toward having a body that is designed to be resilient in the face of stress, including the stress brought about by disease.

How to Build Healthy Habits

When you're in the hospital for a medical intervention, doctors don't necessarily have the time to talk through other important concerns—such as why you should exercise or eat well or sleep more.

And even when you're at an appointment for a routine visit, there's often no mention of the importance of these lifestyle changes. Too often, a medical visit goes something like this: You come in and you're asked to step on a scale. Next, a cuff is tightened around your upper arm and your blood pressure is measured. Then your blood is drawn. All the while, the person who is taking these measurements, who is perfectly pleasant, is scribbling away, barely making eye contact. What happens next is often . . . nothing. If all these measurements and readings are within the normal range, you're told to come back in a year. But if one or more of them are out of range, well, that's when you are told, in so many words, that what you've been doing, how you've been living your life, hasn't been working and now you need to make some changes. For instance, when it comes to blood pressure, we talk about two numbers, systolic and diastolic, written as, for example 120/80 mm Hg. The first number represents the force of the blood flow when it is pumped out of the heart. The second is measured between heartbeats; it is the resting pressure of the blood vessels when the heart is not pumping. Both numbers are important. The American Heart Association notes that almost half of US adults have high blood pressure.

Blood pressure changes throughout the day based on your activities, but medical practitioners use certain guidelines to tell whether an intervention is required. For instance, according to the AHA, hypertension Stage 1 occurs when systolic blood pressure is 130 to 139 or diastolic is 80 to 89. In this range, your healthcare professional should prescribe lifestyle changes. They may consider adding medication based on your risk of heart disease or stroke and should add medication if you have other conditions such as diabetes, heart failure, and kidney disease. In hypertension Stage 2, with systolic levels above 140 or diastolic levels above 90, your healthcare professional should prescribe blood pressure medication and lifestyle changes. In what the AHA calls hypertensive crisis, with numbers over 180 systolic or 120 diastolic, you need immediate medical attention.

The truth is, often but not always, when we get the information that some essential biomarker reading is not where it should be, our body has been grappling with whatever the issue is for quite some time. Getting "dinged" with an out-of-range test result is what finally gives us the chance to evaluate our lifestyle. My job, and the job of my colleagues, is to become better allies for our patients, to truly understand the stress they're under, so we can help them make meaningful, yet realistic, lifestyle choices and changes.

The Healing Power of Resilience

I've thought long and hard about how I can best help my patients, many of whom the mainstream medical community writes off as being "noncompliant" because they don't have either the knowledge or the resources they need to follow a doctor's advice. When the problem can be solved by changing something about the environment or behavior and then the patient seemingly chooses not to change—well, doctors don't like it. This is the sort of "I told you so" attitude that comes about when a doctor does something such as recommend eating less processed foods and more fresh produce, without connecting the dots that the patient eats what they do because of economic limitations, not disobedience. What might look at first glance like a lack of cooperation is an opportunity for a medical expert to help someone learn how to build resilience.

So how can I better help my patients find the resilience they'll need to make the kinds of lifestyle changes that will positively influence their health? First, I've dropped the word *noncompliant* from my vocabulary because it denies that there are likely preexisting or extenuating circumstances that make it hard or impossible for a patient to follow through and change. Life is stressful, and I've found that shaming or blaming patients is, frankly, disrespectful. My job isn't to judge; it's to help my patients understand that by taking control of what they *can*, they may mitigate the harm caused to their bodies by what they *can't*. To do this, I need to partner with my patients and help them understand why certain lifestyle choices may negatively be affecting their health. Once they're aware of the *why*, then we can focus on *how*, and they might begin to modify their behavior, build resilience, and begin a journey toward health.

Changing aspects of one's lifestyle is not easy. Even if we have the resources we need to, say, upgrade our diet from overprocessed fast food to fresh organic whole food (requiring both the physical access to this kind of food and the financial resources to buy it), it's just not that easy to change the way we eat when we've become habituated to eating a certain way. Or we may strive to get more sleep, but our young children and their needs make this difficult or impossible. Any number of factors might make change difficult, and it's important to acknowledge these factors. But that doesn't mean that we just give up. Any change we make, however minor or incremental, matters.

Exercise, nutrition, and sleep are generally understood to be three key lifestyle factors that influence our overall health and well-being. The good news is that it is never too late to improve our behaviors in these macro areas, and even micro or incremental improvements in one area can have a positive effect on our overall health. Below, I've described a few micro improvements to get you thinking about what might be possible in your life.

Nutrition

Our culture, especially our medical culture, uses body mass index (BMI), waist circumference, and weight as important metrics to gauge a person's baseline general health and to predict the development of certain chronic illnesses. Carrying excess body fat affects our biology in many ways. First of all, the additional effort required to maintain and support a larger body puts extra strain on our physiological systems. A larger body mass, especially one that is above the range of what would be considered normal for our individual BMI, requires more energy to maintain basic functions such as breathing, circulation, and digestion. This increased metabolic demand can put additional stress on the body's organs and systems.

A pause here for a quick note on BMI: It is an imperfect tool, and a somewhat controversial one. BMI calculates a ratio of weight to height, providing a single number that places a person on a spectrum of being underweight, normal weight, overweight, or obese. However, this calculation doesn't account for the complexities of human body composition. A professional athlete, for instance, might have a high BMI due to muscle mass, not excess body fat. On the flip side, older adults often lose muscle mass while gaining fat, potentially leading to a normal BMI despite having potentially unhealthy levels of body fat. BMI also doesn't consider factors such as bone density, fat distribution, or ethnic variations in body composition, all of which can influence health outcomes. The focus on a single number can also contribute to weight stigma and body-image issues, potentially leading to unhealthy behaviors. In sum, we are now more conscious of the limitations of BMI as a measurement, but it still has utility, especially when used in conjunction with other metrics that can help us analyze a person's health with regard to their body weight, and that's why I use it here.

Being overweight affects hormone production and regulation and contributes to conditions such as insulin resistance and glucose dysregulation, both of which may lead to the development of type 2 diabetes. It contributes to high blood pressure, high cholesterol, and elevated triglyceride levels, which can, in turn, lead to atherosclerosis (the buildup of plaques in the arteries), which may inhibit blood flow and the heart's ability to function optimally. Carrying excess body fat is also known to increase inflammation, which is a precursor to a whole host of chronic illnesses, including diabetes, heart disease, and some cancers.

Many of us don't know that fat (adipose tissue) is not just clusters of inert cells—it is an independently functioning endocrine organ that interacts with our hormones to affect such things as satiety, insulin sensitivity, and how we metabolize both carbohydrates and fats. When we are chronically obese, often defined in shorthand as having a BMI over 30 (a normal BMI is considered between 18.5 and 25, and overweight

25–30), this can dysregulate our metabolic systems. This chronic metabolic dysregulation, which is a form of chronic stress, contributes to many preventable diseases, such as osteoarthritis, diabetes, coronary artery diseases, and cancer, among others. The physical stress of carrying excess weight can also strain other organs, such as our lungs, gallbladder, and liver, and contribute to disruptive conditions such as sleep apnea and depression. Knowing this may give us the *why* we need so that our desire to lose weight feels more concrete, more medically imperative, and is therefore more likely something that we'll do our best to address.

And as far as the heart goes, Johns Hopkins researchers have shown that excess weight is more than an "accomplice" in the development of heart problems. Extra pounds can directly cause heart-muscle injury. Doctors determined this by studying levels of a cardiac enzyme called troponin, which is released by injured heart-muscle cells. It is commonly used as a determinant of when someone is having a heart attack, but sensitive lab tests can now measure troponin at much lower levels. Johns Hopkins researchers measured the troponin levels as well as BMI of more than ninety-five hundred adults, ages fifty-three to seventy-three, and found that higher BMI was strongly linked to higher troponin levels—and those who were both the most obese and had high troponin levels were nine times more likely to develop heart failure than those who had normal weight and undetectable troponin.

Knowledge is power, but it is not a magic formula. I want to be clear here and say that obesity is a complex and difficult chronic disease to address because it is influenced by so many factors, including socioeconomic, genetic, environmental, and lifestyle.

Conversely, being chronically underweight can also contribute to the onset of chronic diseases. Being underweight is usually a sign of malnourishment, the state in which the body isn't getting the nutrients it needs to function optimally. Malnutrition weakens our bones, our hearts, and deprives our organs of the nutrition they need to operate properly and efficiently. Over time, being severely underweight can also weaken the immune system, lead to heart disease, contribute to the onset of certain types of cancer, and cause depression.

This is why nutrition is so crucial to building physiological resilience. Our body needs to be fueled in ways that promote homeostasis and optimal functionality.

Food is not only what fuels our bodies, but it is also what heals them. To build physiological resilience and experience optimal health, we need these nutritional basics:

- Macronutrients, including protein (from lean-animal or vegetable sources), give the body what it needs to build and repair tissue, keep metabolic systems humming along, keep the immune system strong, and provide the energy the body needs to perform optimally. Along with protein, we need healthy carbohydrates, such as whole grains, fruits, and vegetables, to help with all of the processes mentioned, and also to help regulate blood sugar, keep our digestive system functioning, and build up heart health. Another essential macronutrient is fat, and the best sources of this are the healthy fats found in nuts, seeds, and fruits such as avocado and olive (and their oils), and fish. These essential fats are needed to maintain heart and brain health, facilitate nutrient absorption, balance our hormones, and keep inflammation in check, among other resilience-building things.
- Micronutrients include vitamins and minerals, phytonutrients, and antioxidants. Even though we need these substances only

in relatively tiny amounts, their impact on our health is huge. We need micronutrients for everything from the efficient production of vital substances such as hormones and enzymes, to the proper functioning of our immune system and efficient energy production. Without the right input of micronutrients, we also leave ourselves susceptible to chronic illnesses such as heart disease, degenerative cognitive diseases, and cancers, among others.
- Fiber. The body needs the fiber found in whole grains, vegetables (especially leafy green ones), and fruits to keep our digestive system working efficiently so that the body can best metabolize our nutritional intake.
- Water. We simply can't survive without it. Making sure you get adequate hydration is essential for the body to function and perform at its best. The Mayo Clinic says that means about 15.5 cups of fluids a day for men and 11.5 cups of fluids a day for women.

I don't prescribe any particular diet to patients. The most common diets we talk about in cardiology, though, are plant-based or vegetarian diets, Mediterranean diets, and the DASH diet, which stands for Dietary Approaches to Stop Hypertension, and focuses on fruits and vegetables, whole grains, nuts and seeds, lean proteins, and lowfat dairy. Instead, I often recommend to many of my patients that they meet with a nutritionist, who can take the time to review how and what they are eating and make good recommendations on where to make changes. I also run through the general, simple advice that withstands the test of time and trends: Eat whole foods and avoid processed foods as much as possible, especially those laden with additives, chemicals, salt, and sugar. And do what you can to not overeat. For instance, avoid getting overly hungry. Eat mindfully, meaning avoid snacking when distracted, such as while watching TV or scrolling on your phone. Try to pick filling foods, and wait for a while after eating before going back for seconds. In the words of the inimitable food writer Michael Pollan, "Eat food. Not too much. Mostly plants."

Sleep

We spend roughly one-third of our lives in the dreamy state of sleep, but most of us rarely give it much thought. Sure, we know how rough we can feel—groggy, foggy, or grouchy—if we don't get enough of it. But why is it that we feel poorly if we haven't had a good night's sleep? The overall ennui we feel when we aren't well rested is the body's way of letting us know that we are depriving it of something important, just as being thirsty is the body's way of telling us we need to hydrate. Sleep, in the most simplistic terms, is a process of healing, for both the body and mind. And it's an activity that is essential to building and maintaining biological resilience and warding off illness and disease.

When we don't get enough sleep, our brain (particularly the prefrontal cortex, the area of the brain responsible for many important functions including impulse control, critical thinking, decision-making, recall, and, when working in concert with the limbic system, emotional regulation) can't function optimally. We need to sleep an adequate amount (research is showing that there is a sleep "sweet spot," which is between seven to nine hours a day for most adults) for our brain to process and remove metabolic waste that has built up over our waking day. When we're in the stillness of sleep, our brain cells contract, creating channels that allow cerebrospinal fluid to wash over the brain and flush it of toxins and waste. That's why, when we wake up after a good night's sleep, we feel so refreshed—our brains have literally been cleansed during the night.

Additionally, sleep is the time when the brain consolidates memory and learning, and that's why a test taker is often advised that getting a good night's sleep before an exam is more beneficial than staying up all night cramming.

Just as sleep cleanses and refreshes the brain, the body also benefits from the restorative powers of sleep. While we sleep, our body goes through its own regenerative processes to prepare us to meet the day with resilience. Sleep is a time when our metabolic systems slow and we expend less energy, holding on to the fuel we'll need when it's time again to act. It's also a time of repair for our cells and tissue. When we don't get enough sleep, our immune system may become sluggish, leaving us more vulnerable to getting sick. Along with messing with our metabolic systems, inadequate sleep increases inflammation, which can in turn set us up for making some less than ideal lifestyle choices, such as overindulging in caffeine, sugar, and overprocessed foods, in a vain attempt to perk ourselves up. Most alarming, a lack of sleep—especially chronic sleep deprivation, which is a pernicious form of chronic stress and is perceived by the body as such—contributes to the onset of chronic illnesses such as cardiovascular diseases, diabetes, and cancer.

First of all, sleep lowers our levels of cortisol—one of the key hormones involved in the stress response. When we aren't sleeping enough, our cortisol levels remain higher than they should, leading to all of the stress-related symptoms we have previously discussed. Sleep deprivation is also linked to such issues as depression and anxiety, cognitive issues including difficulty making decisions and solving problems, and difficulty with controlling emotions.

One study about the detrimental effects of sleep deprivation that I find particularly concerning looked at two groups of medical residents: one that was analyzed after being on call for twenty-four hours, and another group evaluated after a normal workday. The two groups were tested for heart-rate variability, cortisol levels, cognitive performance—including reaction time to stimuli—and general mood, based on a self-assessment of sixteen different questions that were evaluated using a ten-level Likert scale. A Likert scale, named after social psychologist Rensis Likert, is often used to evaluate people's attitudes, opinions, or behaviors. This type of survey requires respondents to choose their answer from a spectrum such as strongly agree, agree, neutral, disagree, strongly disagree; or always, often, sometimes, rarely, never. The doctors in the on-call group measured significantly lower than the control group in all measures: physiological, performance, and mood.

If the doctors treating patients are themselves impaired, imagine the impact on quality of care. I think about this study not only from my perspective as a doctor, but also as a cardiologist who knows that long-term sleep deprivation can lead to increased cardiovascular risk. The American Heart Association added sleep as the eighth critical lifestyle factor for cardiovascular well-being when updating its Life Simple 7 recommendations in 2022 to Life's Essential 8.

As you know, I'm fascinated by the heart so I want to share a bit more about how sleep affects it. When we do get adequate sleep, our heart has an important opportunity to work a little less rigorously. Experts are beginning to understand that the natural dip in blood pressure that occurs when we sleep well protects us from developing such things as high blood pressure, coronary artery disease, heart failure, and stroke. Research shows that when an adult over the age of forty-five gets too little or too much sleep (again, anywhere between seven and nine hours is the sweet spot), she doesn't get the benefits of this coronary quieting, and so the body becomes more vulnerable to developing chronic heart diseases.

A final warning: As I mentioned, when we don't get enough sleep and our stress levels remain elevated, our performance—both our cognitive and physical abilities—are adversely affected, often causing our job performance, home life, or our relationships to suffer. A lack of sleep affects us in a multitude of ways.

Some key practices to improve sleep hygiene include the following tips from the Department of Psychiatry and Behavioral Sciences at UC Davis:

- Try to go to bed at the same time every day, even on weekends. Establishing a regular rhythm will improve your sleep cycle.
- Make sure your workout is finished at least four hours before bedtime. Regular exercise improves sleep, but the timing is important.
- Develop sleep rituals that clue your body that it's time to slow for the day. Listening to relaxing music, deep-breathing exercises, or drinking caffeine-free tea can be great ways to wind down. On that note, be sure to stay away from caffeine—and alcohol—at least four to six hours before bed.
- Make sure your bedroom is quiet, dark, and comfortable. A cooler room—at about sixty-eight degrees—is optimal for sleep for most people. Blackout shades or curtains or a sleep mask can help create a light-free environment. If noise is a problem, wear earplugs or try white noise or soft, soothing music.
- And lastly, avoid blue light from devices as you wind down for the day. Use a blue-light filter or blue-light-blocking glasses

when looking at screens and do your best to avoid any screens without filters for two hours before sleeping. Or even better, keep screens out of the bedroom entirely. That way you will be less tempted to use them.

Many life stressors can make getting good, quality sleep hard, but sleep is one of the lifestyle factors that can make or break our health. Once we know about the ways we can make a difference in our behaviors, we can start to use them to bolster our Resilience Response. But making lasting lifestyle changes can often be challenging.

Why Are Habits So Hard to Change?

I've described a lot of behaviors above, some of which you might engage in already, and others you hope to adopt as new habits.

A habit is a repetitive behavior that we engage in when we are triggered by something—and that something can be a positive or negative. Habits can be healthy (walking every morning) or unhealthy (smoking), but in both cases, we experience some kind of chemical reward (a runner's high, or the relaxing chemical effects of nicotine). When we engage in these activities regularly and over time, they become encoded in our brains and often become unconscious. Think of someone who chronically bites their nails or someone who automatically takes the same route to work every morning. The more we engage in the behavior, however, the more this process becomes harder and harder to break over time, which can be a negative thing or a positive one. A study on habit formation published in the journal *Psychology, Health & Medicine* in 2011 found that once automaticity had developed, people felt that the behavior—in this case, one of ten simple diet and activity changes designed to help participants lose weight—became "second nature," "worming their way into your brain," and participants noted they "felt quite strange" if they did not do them.

There are three stages when we actively set out to form a positive new habit. It begins with an initiation phase, when the new behavior is identified along with the context in which we will perform it. Next comes the learning phase, during which the behavior is repeated within the context, strengthening the context-behavior association. A simple checklist for self-monitoring can help with this. Last comes the stability phase, when the habit has formed and stuck, so that it has staying power that requires little effort or deliberation.

The way to begin to change or dismantle a habit is to understand that this powerful process must be undone. In these cases, once the brain has strengthened this context-behavior association over time, it will take attention and time to rewire it.

This is why it's important to understand how difficult it is to lose weight when one is suffering from chronic obesity: So many factors are at play—environmental, social, emotional, and physical—that it's difficult for the body to reset in a meaningful, lasting way. And this is why the medical establishment is finally beginning to treat obesity like the chronic disease that it is. The understanding that lifestyle change alone may not be enough to reverse it has ushered in a period of exciting breakthroughs in using medical interventions (such as gastric bypass or the new class of drugs called glucagon-like peptide-1 receptor agonists, known as GLP-1s) to favorably influence metabolic and biological processes. I recently heard a fascinating interview with Dr. Ania Jastreboff, endocrinologist and director of the Yale Obesity Research Center. In a follow-up article, she mentioned the "many barriers to treating obesity, including access, cost, and the stigma, bias, shame, and blame." She made a passionate case for treating patients with obesity the same way doctors treat any patient with a chronic disease, and to use all options available to address it.

Even with helpful medical interventions, it can still be difficult in the long term to change behaviors that can contribute to obesity or other chronic stress-related conditions, as the brain is wired to default back to the unhealthy pattern we had developed over a much-longer time. To make lasting, meaningful change, we need to understand what's driving our behavior in the first place, which means learning to identify the true stressors in our lives. We might be sleeping poorly because we are suspicious that our partner is having an affair, or because our child is being bullied at school. We might find we are stress eating at work to manage having an oppressive boss. Once we've identified those triggers, we can make better-informed decisions about how best to manage them.

For example, some people overeat in response to a stressful event, as stress activates systems associated with metabolism and reward. As we know, during a stressful event the body releases cortisol. If cortisol levels are elevated for a prolonged period, this can lead to increased food consumption, fat storage, and weight gain. Someone who regularly overeats after stress as an unconscious way to self-soothe will likely experience weight gain. Knowing that this habit may lead to these health problems gives us the *why* we need to replace the habit. But first, we may need to explore why we over-eat, and this may mean enlisting the right kind of support, such as confiding in a family member, friend, or a therapist. I am a huge advocate for mental-health treatment and therapy, and believe most of us could benefit from this type of support. I believe we need a medical establishment that works hand in hand with mental-health care—a world in which psychology practices could be built into so many of our medical practices, so we can truly treat the patient as a whole person.

Though I am keenly aware that, unfortunately, my ability to help outside of the doctor's office is limited, I routinely ask my patients if they're depressed, anxious, or have any other psychological concerns when they come to me for an appointment. If they respond yes, I refer them to a specialist who can help them find the right kind of treatment. This is so important to consider when we are dealing with a diagnosis that affects a key organ such as the heart. A statement entitled "Psychological Health, Well-Being, and the Mind-Heart-Body-Connection," released by the American Heart Association in 2021 made clear "there are good data showing clear associations between psychological health and CVD (cardiovascular disease) risk." This is a paradigm-shifting acknowledgment of the mind-body continuum, especially when considering chronic disease and specifically cardiovascular diseases. The statement encourages cardiologists and all healthcare providers to include an assessment of a patient's mental health to get a full understanding of the stressors at play. When I see people in my office, I am always mindful of the ways our mental and physical health are entwined, and I do my best to ensure that my patients are being cared for in body, mind, and spirit.

That's why it's so crucial that we be good to ourselves while we're working to change a habit to better support our health. Changing a habit is rarely a linear process, as Andy and so many of my patients can attest to—often we get stuck at stage one or stage two or need to adjust our goal or our context. While doing so, we need to refrain from judging ourselves harshly or beating ourselves up when we face the inevitable roadblock or setback.

Learning to nurture our body in ways that promote its inherent, biological resilience is the work of a lifetime. It entails learning how to assess habits and behaviors we may never before have examined, and finding the resources we need to modify and change them. This kind of positive adjustment can be something as simple as reaching for a bottle of water instead of a can of diet soda; taking a quick walk when we feel distracted rather than scrolling on social media; acknowledging discomfort when it arises in an interaction with someone and approaching it with curiosity rather than fear or judgment. Every time we make this kind of choice, we signal to both our body and brain that there is a different, healthier way of doing things. It's never an all-or-nothing proposition—life just isn't like that. It's a fluid process, this learning to build and sustain our health, and one that can give us a new sense of how capable we are of meeting life's challenges.

No one exemplifies this truth better than Gabby Giffords, a former congresswoman.

On January 8, 2011, in Tucson, Arizona, while hosting a "Congress on Your Corner" event in the parking lot of a supermarket, forty-year-old congresswoman Gabby Giffords was shot in the head at point-blank range in what has been described as an assassination attempt, but which was, in fact, a mass shooting; six people were killed that day, including a nine-year-old girl. Giffords and twelve others were injured.

Giffords was rushed to the Medical Center of Tucson in critical condition and put in the ICU. There, part of her skull was removed to relieve pressure on her brain. Hospital spokespeople were clear about the severity of her injury, stating that 95 percent of victims of this type of traumatic brain injury do not survive. The other 5 percent remain severely impaired. In just a few days, Gifford was transferred to the Neuroscience Intensive Care Unit at Memorial Hermann-Texas Medical Center in Houston, Texas, where her condition was downgraded from critical to serious. She was then moved to TIRR Memorial Hermann rehabilitation hospital.

Get Fit

There, Gifford was surrounded by what Chief Medical Officer Gerard Francisco has described as an "orchestra" of experts that worked in concert to create a unique treatment plan for her rehabilitation, which was intensive. Giffords had to relearn to speak and was unable to walk unaided. She also had to relearn how to write and relearn many basic activities of daily living. Every day involved hours of speech therapy, occupational therapy, and physical therapy. It was slow, grueling work, but Giffords, who has been described by those around her as an incredibly "bright light," modeled unbelievable resilience as she worked—and continues to work—on recovering. Returning to the elements of the Resilience Response we've explored so far, it's clear that Giffords was modeling each and every one of them: acceptance of her situation; a flexible mindset allowing for change; and a focus on restoring physical health. Just six months after the shooting, she made her first public appearance when she attended a ceremony at Space Center Houston, where her husband of four years, retired astronaut Mark Kelly, was awarded a Space Flight Medal. This marked the beginning of her remarkable return to public life.

In 2013, not long after the Sandy Hook Elementary School gun massacre, Giffords and Kelly founded an organization whose mission is to free our country from the gun violence epidemic. Next, in 2017, Giffords, and her longtime speech therapist, Fabiane "Fabi" Hirsch Kruse, along with Suzy Gershman, founded Friends of Aphasia, an Arizona-based advocacy group whose mission is to restore quality of life to people with aphasia, and to educate and support their friends and family.

I had the chance to interview Gabby in 2022, a little more than a decade after she was shot. Although she is no longer Congresswoman Giffords, her devotion to public service and to improving the lives of others is undiminished—it just looks far different from what she ever could have imagined.

Here's the phrase from our interview that I keep coming back to, year after year: "No matter what, we are resilient. We can be knocked down, and we can rise up."

The physical work that Giffords had to undertake to reach her new normal was enormous. In Giffords's case, however, she could not have become the powerful advocate that she is without the rehabilitation program where she was a patient after being shot.

In some ways, rehab facilities are the perfect place to build new healthy habits: They provide support, accountability, and medical oversight while patients try new behaviors. Rehab facilities don't just help patients get physically back on track, but in the case of cardiac rehabilitation programs help to prevent future heart problems, too. Cardiac rehabilitation programs usually last about three months but can range from two to eight months, but the benefits can last a lifetime. Consider that around eight hundred thousand people in the United States have a heart attack every year—and one in four of those people have had a previous heart attack. Studies have found that cardiac rehabilitation decreases the chance that you will die in the five years following a heart attack or bypass surgery by about 35 percent.

The CDC notes that cardiac rehabilitation can have many physical and mental-health benefits in both the short and long term, including relieving symptoms such as chest pain and helping to build healthier habits such as getting more physical activity, quitting smoking, and eating a heart-healthy diet. The mental benefits of rehab programs are also significant, as it has been proven that people are more likely to feel depressed after a heart attack. Cardiac rehabilitation programs have been shown to help prevent or lessen depression.

Get Fit

Patients who have access to a formal cardiac rehabilitation program are more likely to take their medications, actively make health-promoting lifestyle changes, and, importantly, overcome the fear brought on by the medical trauma they experienced. A well-designed cardiac rehabilitation program addresses the barriers that need to be overcome for a patient to recover and regain both psychological and physical resilience.

Clearly, focusing on lifestyle habits and practices that nourish the body—exercise, nutrition, sleep—are critical not only to helping prevent disease but also to helping us move forward when diagnosed with a disease or illness. One of the most daunting hurdles as we do so is fear. Which brings us to the next aspect of the Resilience Response.

CHAPTER 6

Face Your Fear

We all know what it feels like to be intensely afraid. Our hearts race as our pulse begins to quicken, we start to sweat, we might feel woozy or dizzy, we have an impulse to scream out or to run for the hills or to freeze on the spot. A more subtle form of fear might make us feel nauseated, or nervous. So what happens when we become afraid of something that we've been told we should do, that is supposed to make us healthier? I'm referring, in this instance, to the proven fact that people who have had a heart attack often experience fear that it might happen again. How are they supposed to test their hearts by exerting them through exercise when they are gripped by this thought?

A headline from the American Heart Association sums up the larger issue neatly: "Fear of another heart attack may be a major source of ongoing stress for survivors." A 2024 study found that survivors of an acute heart attack (also called a myocardial infarction, or MI) experienced persistent fear of recurrence following the event. Among the key takeaways from this study were that fear of another heart attack was still significant at follow-up around eight months.

Also, controlling for depression and anxiety, which are common after a heart attack, "did not reduce the impact of fear of recurrence on illness perception and perceived stress from six months to about eight months following the initial event."

This fear of having another MI was persistent and long-lasting, not passing or momentary. So how are heart attack survivors who are intensely afraid of another MI supposed to reengage in life generally and, more specifically, in exercise, one of the very activities that affects their heart, albeit in a positive way?

Interestingly, if you think about the signs of fear that I just listed above, several of them—such as perspiring and increased heart rate—naturally occur not only when we are scared, but also when we are exercising. This starts to make some sense if you remember that exercise is a kind of good stress that challenges the body in ways that help it become stronger and more resilient. A recent study conducted by Michael Otto, PhD, a professor of psychology at Boston University, and Dr. Jasper Smits, director of the Anxiety Research and Treatment Program at Southern Methodist University in Dallas, showed that workouts can help people avoid panic. Sixty volunteers prone to anxiety who took part in a two-week exercise program showed marked improvement in their anxiety sensitivity compared to a control group. "Exercise in many ways is like exposure treatment," says Smits. "People learn to associate the symptoms with safety instead of danger." Though the fear described in the post-MI patients above is distinct from the anxiety experienced by the subjects in Smits and Otto's study, perhaps we can glean some helpful hints on how to slowly, gradually help heart attack survivors work through their fears of recurrence, using appropriate physical exertion.

In some ways this approach is akin to exposure theory, which has been with us since ancient times but experienced a resurgence in the

1950s when psychodynamic theories helped us to begin to understand why it actually works. When faced with something frightening, people often resort to avoidance. While this may offer temporary relief, it ultimately reinforces the fear and prevents us from overcoming it. Exposure therapy aims to break this cycle of avoidance and fear by placing a person in a safe and controlled environment where a therapist gradually exposes them to the object, activity, or situation that causes them fear. This repeated exposure, while initially anxiety provoking, helps the person learn to tolerate and eventually overcome their fear. This approach is not appropriate in all situations (for instance, for some after an acute trauma), but it has been scientifically proven effective and valuable for a range of issues including phobias, panic disorder, social-anxiety disorder, obsessive-compulsive disorder, post-traumatic stress disorder, and generalized anxiety disorder. And as for how exposure therapy works—it's a bit like a reversing or unwinding of the way that habit forming works in the brain: disconnecting or unencoding the trigger from the response, a breaking of the bond between the object or situation that incites the response and the physical response that it creates.

You may have heard the famous words of President Franklin D. Roosevelt from his inaugural address in 1933, "the only thing we have to fear is fear itself." We tend to think of being afraid as somehow a sign of weakness, a feeling we're somehow supposed to avoid or, when it does strike, we're supposed to minimize it and move on from it fast. In truth, being afraid isn't a sign of weak character; it is a healthy instinctual response that's wired into us and that is designed to help us survive.

Fear arises when we encounter anything that threatens our safety and well-being. It is one of the most primal and potent triggers of the stress response, and it has both an emotional component and a physiological component. As psychologist and renowned expert on emotions and nonverbal communication Paul Ekman notes, fear also has three distinguishing elements—Intensity: How severe is the harm that is threatened? Timing: Is the harm immediate or impending? Coping: What, if any, actions can be taken to reduce or eliminate the threat? Are we being chased by a lion or being yelled at by a pissed-off driver in the next lane?

As our bodies and minds size up danger, the amygdala, the brain's fear center, triggers a cascade of neural and hormonal responses. These responses help prepare us for the classic fight, flight, or freeze responses. Our heart rate increases, our muscles tense, our nonessential systems (such as digestion) slow. Our brain may even tune out certain stimuli: This is called cognitive narrowing, when the brain prioritizes immediate survival needs by blocking less urgent input. This can show up as tunnel vision, when our field of visual focus narrows to center on the perceived threat, making it difficult to perceive peripheral stimuli. Intense fear can also overwhelm other cognitive processes, making it difficult to think rationally or make clear decisions, and impairs cognitive functions such as attention, memory, and higher-order thinking. In essence, during fear the brain prioritizes immediate survival mechanisms that help us in the goal of escaping or fighting back against a real or perceived threat.

That's why, when we're surprised or overwhelmed (the weightless plunge of a high roller coaster comes to mind), we may shriek, cover our eyes, or grab hold of the person next to us. But once the threat passes (phew, the ride is over and we're coasting to a stop), our fear dissipates and our brain activity returns to a more neutral state. We can now relax and homeostasis returns. It's like a flare going up from a boat in distress: The signal is seen, the coast guard responds, and all are rescued and brought to shore safely. That said, fear exists on a continuum. Dr. Ekman plots out that from least intense to most intense, we can experience a range of fear from nervousness, to dread, desperation, panic, horror, and, at its most extreme, terror.

So what, exactly, is the difference between fear and stress? Psychologists differentiate between them in the following way: Fear arises when we sense a threat; it is an *immediate response* to actual or perceived danger. Stress can then follow from fear; it is a *physical and psychological response* to demands or pressure. Both fear and stress can be incited by triggers both real and imagined. It's one thing if fear and stress are triggered by a bear crashing through the forest running after you; it's another if you feel that a bear is going to jump out of the woods every time you walk the dog in your local park.

The first is rational; the second less so. So what if the lines between rational and irrational fears grow blurry? What if we're so overcome with fear that a return to a sense of safety feels impossible? Or, worse, what if our fear doesn't dissipate, and it affects our ability to take adequate care of ourselves? When this happens, we can become paralyzed; it can be difficult or even impossible for us to continue to take the actions we need to protect and promote our health and well-being. For instance, if someone has suffered a heart attack, it can be scary to start an exercise regimen, even though this is an essential ingredient in helping their heart become more healthy.

In my practice I see this too often, unfortunately, in the wake of a scary medical incident. I think back to my twenty-seven-year-old patient Miriam, who came to me with shortness of breath and with severe heart palpitations in the wake of her father's death. What she was actually suffering from was a series of panic attacks. Miriam's fear caused her to experience real symptoms.

Research psychologist Kelly McGonigal talks about how we can recognize and harness fear before it leads to a response like Miriam's.

The Healing Power of Resilience

During an NPR interview with Guy Raz that aired in August of 2019, she told him that she was experiencing the physiological changes brought on by stress as they spoke. He asked her to describe them. "I would describe them as changes that are taking place in my brain and body to help me rise to a moment that matters." She went on, "So I'm feeling alert. I'm feeling a bit raw and vulnerable, as if I'm more open to the world around me. And I can sense my heart beating. It's not racing. But I definitely feel—I sense this type of stress as a surge of energy that is encouraging me to engage." The challenge of managing one's fear to speak in public isn't the same as that of managing one's fear after a loss or when facing the diagnosis of a chronic or severe illness, but what they do have in common is that they point back to the need to rely on our resilience: the innate ability each of us has to meet life's challenges and take the next right action. We can be afraid but still go on. Which is why it's a crucial step in a Resilience Response.

But when we cannot muster a Resilience Response in these situations, fear can be corrosive. Being constantly fearful brings on the same physiological and psychological reactions as chronic stress: If fear persists, it can impact the body's ability to regain homeostasis, and all the side effects that brings, and also erode a person's sense of agency. Take, for example, the fear of having a heart attack—also known as cardiophobia. As I mentioned, it can interfere with one's ability to engage in heart-healthy activities, such as exercise, as the sufferer fears this may trigger a cardiac event. Acute cardiophobia is rare, but those who suffer from it can actually experience some of the physical symptoms of a heart attack—such as heart palpitations or shortness of breath—but show no medical evidence of heart problems.

Fear can lead to even more extreme consequences, too. In some cases, fear can cause the chambers of the heart to "vibrate" (ventricular fibrillation) in ways that interfere with the heart's ability to pump blood efficiently. Walter Cannon, the renowned physiologist, gave this kind of psychosomatic cardiac arrest the spooky name *voodoo death*.

That's one example of how what we think can affect how we feel, both psychologically and physically. The late Martin Samuels, a neurologist at Brigham and Women's Hospital in Boston, was renowned for his work on how the brain influences cardiac health. Samuel's pioneering work in what has become known as the field of neurocardiology focused on the interplay between the nervous system (the brain) and the cardiovascular system (the heart). His work and the work of other neurocardiologists is built on the understanding that the functionality of the brain and heart are intertwined, and that stress and fear can have a demonstrably costly effect on the structural integrity of the cardiovascular system, including the heart.

Samuels and his team gathered case studies of people who died suddenly when an overwhelming surge of stress chemicals caused cardiac malfunction. While it doesn't happen often, the unexpected and overwhelming rush of adrenaline brought on by an overwhelming emotional shock—especially fear—can cause the heart to seize and stop. We can actually be scared to death. Usually there is an underlying condition in these cases (such as heart disease), but not always.

Sometimes, it's not necessarily fear that incites a suddenly fatal response. There are also cases of people whose hearts give out when they're overwhelmed with positive excitement, such as when their team wins a major sporting event. One of the memorable cases Samuels often mentioned was that of a man who died suddenly after hitting a hole in one while playing golf. He made the shot, walked up to the cup, retrieved his ball, then turned to his friend and said, "Wow. I just hit a hole in one. I can die now." And he did. Right there on the golf course in front of his friend.

The Healing Power of Resilience

President Franklin D. Roosevelt's words around being afraid of fear actually feel useful when you consider that many of the chemicals released in our brains and bodies when we feel fear are the same ones released when we are animated by a sudden positive feeling. That quickening feeling presages an excitement that could be either good or bad. The key players are the same and include dopamine, norepinephrine, and epinephrine (or adrenaline).

The two responses, fear and excitement, also involve some of the same brain structures. For instance, the amygdala plays a key role in the emotional processing of fear and anxiety. But it also interacts with the reward system, influencing how we learn to recognize and how we remember both adverse and pleasurable experiences.

The specific combination and levels of these neurochemicals, the neural pathways they activate, and the context and our interpretation of the situation all work together to determine the resulting emotion. The challenge and the opportunity are to realize this and work to consciously harness this unexpected burst of "energy" for positive purposes rather than negative ones.

I have seen firsthand how managing fear in the face of a cardiac event or illness will inform the level of one's health and well-being going forward. I recently saw a postmenopausal woman, Cathy, in her fifties, who is a professor of English literature at a local university. I'd sent her for a screening for heart disease, based on her family history, and her calcium score indicated that she had heart disease. A calcium score is determined by using a noninvasive, specialized CT scan to measure the calcium deposits in the coronary arteries, which reflects the extent of plaque buildup. A score of 0 indicates no detectable calcified plaque and a very low risk of cardiovascular disease events in the next several years. A score between 1 and 10 suggests low cardiovascular risk, while scores between 11 and 100 indicate moderate cardiovascular risk, and above 100, significant risk. The calcium score doesn't directly measure the degree of artery blockage, but it is a useful tool for measuring risk of cardiac events.

When Cathy came back in for her follow-up visit and I shared with her that her numbers indicated elevated risk, she immediately panicked and asked, "Am I going to die?"

Cathy was scared. I had to reassure her that, no, this was not a death sentence. But that it did mean she would need to make some lifestyle changes. We started discussing her diet and exercise habits. I also told her that it was completely normal that she might feel afraid right now. When my patients are afraid, one of the first things I do is validate the fear response. I let them know they are normal for being afraid as, in many cases, they just survived a trauma, for instance, a heart surgery, procedure, or new diagnosis. I find it's important to say this to them, and often I see relief on their faces. Most have never been told that a change in medical status or a diagnosis is legitimately experienced as a trauma, so giving them this understanding helps. Once we establish that, we can then work on how to face their fear.

In this instance, I asked Cathy if she felt that she had adequate emotional support to help her digest and accept this news. I was relieved when she told me she was meeting her sister right after our appointment. I talked about how good it was that we'd caught the problem early and that I felt confident that she would be able to make the adjustments she needed to live a full and rich life with heart disease. This seemed to reassure her a bit, and she began to ask me good questions, which signaled to me that she was already beginning to move through her fear. I tell my patients that knowing they have heart disease is a good thing—because only then can we deal with it and get them the proper treatment or look for the correct pathway to hopefully prevent an event such as a heart attack. Essentially, we begin on the road of managing the condition like a chronic disease, rather than a sudden catastrophe.

I'm a huge believer that knowledge is power—especially in managing chronic heart disease—and so with Cathy we talked about the research that might be helpful to her treatment. I was glad that she was seeing her sister soon, but I mentioned how important it is to have emotional support at a time such as this, and that this might include seeing a therapist if her fear escalated or did not subside. I shared how data shows how calming activities, such as meditating or deep breathing, are incredibly effective at transforming or neutralizing fear, and she casually mentioned that this might be the moment for deepening her yoga practice. I wholeheartedly agreed. I felt reassured that, by the time she left my office, she was already working on healthy and resilient strategies for working with her fear, rather than letting it overwhelm her. I just saw her in my office, one year to the day of her heart disease diagnosis. She was back at work, thriving in her teaching, no longer paralyzed by fear but facing her new life head-on.

Moving Through Fear

Fear is often the first signal that an event might be challenging. It alerts us to potential dangers or obstacles. It prompts us to evaluate potential risks and to consider the consequences of what we might do next. We then have to assess our potential courses of action. Courage, I believe, isn't the absence of fear, but the ability to acknowledge fear and confront it. It's about choosing a course of action despite our fear, making choices based on our values and goals, even when those choices are difficult or uncertain.

Face Your Fear

One of the ways you can measure the success of the Resilience Response in the wake of a major health event such as a heart attack is to note the choices someone makes afterward.

This kind of event gives us the rare opportunity to reevaluate our lives. I have had patients express a deepening appreciation for being alive, and for having the chance to make changes that will allow them to live more fully and authentically. I've had patients quit jobs they hate, decide to marry their longtime partner, go for it and have another child, decide to move closer to family—in short to make all kinds of positive life changes, all of which they say they would not have had *the courage* to make if they hadn't experienced the fear brought on by a health crisis.

As former Navy SEAL commander Rich Diviney says, "Fear serves a distinct purpose: It allows us to recognize, understand, and assess risk. To be fearless means that we are ignoring those cues—rushing into risk without considering the consequences. Courage requires more strength because it is, quite literally, the act of stepping into our fear. . . . There is a predetermined level where fear starts to kick in, and it varies from person to person. In other words, some people start to feel fear before others might, and vice versa. Courage, as an attribute, speaks to how efficiently and frequently we are able to step into our fear. The good news is we can increase our level of courage."

That's good news, because the truth is, simply being alive takes courage. Every day, every one of us is called upon to show up in the world, despite how scared we may feel at that moment. For example, after a bad car crash, it can be difficult to get behind the wheel again. Or it can be even more specific: If we were attacked by someone wearing a red jacket, the sight of anyone wearing that color will draw our eye and may elicit irrational fear. Or, as I've mentioned, after a major health event or the onset of a chronic disease, it can be difficult to know how to move through the world. It can feel absolutely contraindicated to someone who has coronary artery disease or another heart issue to put further stress on the heart by consciously engaging in activities that will elevate their heart rate. I often hear things like "But hasn't my heart been injured? Shouldn't I give it a rest?" But every time we do show up, face our fear, and make courageous choices, we're building resilience.

Resilience, when we frame it this way—as Dr. Valentin Fuster, physician-in-chief of Mount Sinai Hospital and president of the Fuster Heart Hospital of Mount Sinai, recently described it—is not a return to a former state. The fear is still there. It's about moving forward by actively pushing against challenges rather than capitulating to feelings of despair. He likened this to "swimming against the current," which takes, you guessed it, courage. This is one of my favorite definitions of resilience because it's based on *action*. It's an important reminder that resilience is a practice, a thing that we do when we are faced with stress.

It is normal, after diagnosis, to be afraid. You might be consumed by questions such as: Will this treatment work? Will the disease progress rapidly? Will I still be able to do the things I love? But trying to manage this fear while hanging on to our hopes and expectations for the future can be challenging and make it difficult for us to retain perspective and a healthy outlook on life.

As a cardiologist, every day I encounter patients who grapple with the fear that comes with a hard diagnosis. When I tell a young mother that she's in the early stages of heart disease, or I am working with a patient who has just survived his second heart attack, I make space for the fear that naturally arises. Often at this moment patients acutely feel their inevitable mortality. This reality is perhaps the scariest thing that we humans encounter. These moments are difficult, painful, and quite natural, and it's paramount that my patients feel safe, respected, and seen when this fear arises. Palliative-care physician BJ Miller, whose story we encountered earlier in this book, calls this kind of mortal fear "the mother of all fears" because it doesn't come from an external threat—it comes from our inner awareness that we simply cannot escape death.

Miller talks passionately about the opportunities this fear offers: It can give us clarity about what matters most to us; it can facilitate a new appreciation for life; or it may give us a sense of life's fleeting beauty. Embracing this fear is not easy. Miller recommends we approach our fear with respect and with awareness of how it informs our sense of our vulnerability. He talks about learning to "dance" with fear, and we can begin to do this by acknowledging fear as a natural part of life. When we allow space for our fear around illness, disability, or even death, we're honoring the reality of the human condition—and our mortality and our limited time on earth—in ways that ultimately allow us to choose to live a more meaningful, more heartfelt life, thereby making the most of the time that we are here.

Coming face-to-face with our fear of death is a bracing, often transformative moment for my patients, so I choose my words carefully. Once the diagnosis is made known, and some basic questions have been answered, I follow my patient's lead on where we go next. I need to make space so my patient can digest what is often a profound and certainly a scary change in their health status. When they are ready, then we'll work together to build a treatment plan that acknowledges their fear while putting into place a comprehensive program that will help them build their resilience, maintain their health, and, importantly, help them restore a sense of well-being.

That's what Chris and I did. Chris, in his mid-fifties, is my brother-in-law. He and my husband grew up in the wilds of upstate New York, where Chris still lives. He's a big, strong guy who works in construction and spends his free time outdoors hunting and fishing.

Last fall, Chris trekked out into the ancient evergreen forest that meets his property. An avid hunter and experienced outdoorsman, he often goes deer hunting by himself. That particular morning, he woke up feeling a bit stiff and out of sorts, so he took some aspirin before he left the house. But once he was deep in the woods, he suddenly felt tired and a bit dizzy, so he turned around and headed home. When he got there, he was gripped by a tightness in his chest. "Something's not right," he told his partner. She immediately called 911 and EMS promptly arrived, loaded him into their vehicle, and whisked him off to the local hospital.

Preliminary blood work showed that his cardiac enzyme levels were high, which is an indicator of heart injury. He was rushed to the cardiac-catheterization lab, where imaging showed that he had a tight blockage in the proximal or very beginning portion of his LAD (left anterior descending) artery, the coronary artery that supplies 50 percent of the blood to the heart muscle. When this artery is fully blocked, the resulting heart attack is known as the widow-maker, due to how lethal it can be.

Fortunately for Chris, his heart function remained normal even though he had experienced a significant heart attack. With a relatively strong, intact heart and because his artery was not fully blocked, Chris was able to avoid major surgery. He was treated with a stent insertion: A catheter was inserted into the artery and a stent was placed inside it to open the blockage and restore blood flow. Afterward he was kept in the hospital for a few days, and his treatment protocol was drawn up. He would be put on aspirin, a second blood thinner, a statin to lower his cholesterol levels, and blood pressure medicine. He was also asked to monitor his blood pressure and make important lifestyle changes that would better support his heart health.

Chris, the father of a beloved teenage daughter, took this wake-up call seriously. He immediately began to make significant adjustments to his lifestyle, including modifying his diet, lowering his sodium intake, and eating less game and meat, among other things; taking daily walks; and faithfully taking his medication. By Christmastime, when I last saw him, he looked great. In only a few short months, he'd lost about thirty pounds and he looked healthier than he had in years. But there was one thing he wasn't yet able to overcome: He told me that despite knowing that a stent was in place keeping his artery open and his heart functioning, and he was taking medications and following a diet that, taken together, would further lower his risk of developing more atherosclerosis (the buildup of plaque in the arteries), he was terrified about going out into the woods by himself, convinced that he'd have another heart attack and die out there alone.

I told Chris this level of fear is to be expected because having a major health crisis, such as a heart attack, is an acute trauma, and that like all traumatic experiences this would need to be worked through. To this end, talking about his fear was the first and most important step. I was glad he felt comfortable sharing his fear with me, and I also suggested that he might want to see a therapist if the fear persisted. More than anything else, I told him to give himself time.

I know the wilderness is his sanctuary, and I could see how hard this was for him. "What if you just go stand by the edge of the woods, just to get in touch with the trees and the smell and the quiet?" I offered. He hugged me and promised me he'd see what he could do.

After the holidays were over, we checked in with each other regularly. He told me that when he'd go out for his daily walk, he'd go to the edge of his property and then walk along it, adjacent to the forest. Then, after a few days of this, he was able step a bit deeper into the woods, reminding himself that he was now in better shape than he was a few months ago, and that his heart condition was being treated and monitored. After a while, he was able to go a bit farther, and each time he ventured farther and farther, until one day he just found himself walking in the woods, his dog by his side, no longer consumed by the fear that had gripped him for so many months. Chris was, step by step, "dancing" with his fear, and by being willing to do this, he was not only rebuilding his heart health, but also building his resilience.

I admire Chris for taking the time he needed to find his way back to what he loved. I recently learned that he was practicing his own unique version of exposure therapy, taking baby steps back into an activity he once loved. It's something we all can try: wading into safe, shallow water after a scary incident in the waves. Or trying something new by confronting a tenacious fear or phobia. For instance, for someone afraid of dogs, they might start with minimal exposure, such as watching brief videos where dogs are positively portrayed. Then they could graduate to observing live dogs in person from a safe distance, and, eventually, with the help of a trusted friend or professional, to interacting with calm, well-behaved dogs in controlled settings. In Chris's case, he was doing a bit of both: making his way back to doing what he loved while managing the ongoing fear that his heart might fail him. The last time I checked in with him, we didn't even touch on his health (which is now quite good), and this was the clearest indication to me that he had, quite successfully, overcome his fear. For me, this is what it's all about: helping people get back to enjoying what they love about life—and not allowing a health event to take that away.

But What About Anxiety?

I've mentioned anxiety a few times in this chapter, but in some ways it's not like fear at all—it's another problem entirely.

Put a different way, anxiety is a chronic, lower-grade fear (on the spectrum from nervousness to terror) related to our perception of whether we'll be equipped to meet and respond to future life stressors. But just because it's lower grade doesn't mean not to take it seriously: Anxiety can be especially pernicious when we're faced with a health issue. But worries may show up in areas of our life besides health that we had otherwise assumed were secure. We may need to take time off from work or even rethink what we do for work if we're faced with limitations on our mobility or our energy levels. Our financial security may be threatened if we're faced with unexpected or ongoing medical bills. We may need more physical and emotional support from our friends and loved ones, and this may cause us to worry, too, especially if we've been used to going it alone.

The American psychologist David Barlow, an expert on anxiety disorders, succinctly defines anxiety as "the fear of fear." He means by this that unlike fear, which is a response to a real, immediate threat, anxiety is an abstract, anticipatory form of stress that focuses on a nonexistent fear and therefore triggers the same reactions in our mind and body as fear. What makes anxiety so difficult to treat is the intangible nature of these fear-inducing thoughts. And as an anxious person is stuck in a flight, fight, or freeze response, that strengthens the perceived validity of their anxious beliefs. In other words, and to make this less abstract, people with debilitating anxiety become trapped in a mindset that tells them that because they feel frightened when they think about some future event or outcome, this feeling (which can manifest emotionally, physically, or both) must mean their anxiety is justified.

How do we manage the natural, very human experience of anxiety in a way that fortifies us, rather than harms us?

I recently had the chance to speak with Robert Leahy, director of the American Institute for Cognitive Therapy in New York, about the importance of resilience in combating both fear and anxiety. "I love the concept of resilience because it embraces the inevitable hardships and challenges of life in a way that expands our awareness that hardship—and the tough emotions that come with it—is inevitable." He goes on to say, "Once we accept the reality that life is sometimes hard, we can adjust our mindset accordingly, embrace all of our feelings, and meet life's challenges from a place of integrity and strength." We talked about how a resilient mindset allows us to look at our fear or manage our anxiety, knowing that life is all about change. Accepting, sitting with, and moving through discomfort allows us to keep making choices based on our values and goals, knowing that the only true constant in life is change.

One effective way to combat chronic anxiety is cognitive behavioral therapy. CBT is built upon the belief that our interpretations of events, rather than the events themselves, influence our emotional responses. In CBT a therapist and a client work together to identify and challenge negative thought patterns, replacing them with more balanced and realistic perspectives. This leads to changes in behavior and gradually confronting triggers in order to reduce anxiety. CBT teaches practical problem-solving skills and coping mechanisms such as relaxation techniques and mindfulness.

One example is a written CBT exercise called the Thought Record, which asks us to examine an action that made us uncomfortable or worried, and why it incited certain feelings or reactions. The exercise first asks us to write down what the situation was. Consider one that typically triggers anxiety for you, such as giving a presentation at a conference. Next, identify and record the automatic thoughts and behaviors this situation conjures up. Things like "I'm going to mess up; everyone will judge me; I've never been good at public speaking; I am going to embarrass myself." Next, consider the evidence for and against the thoughts. Things like "I messed up the last time" or "I forget things when I'm in front of a crowd," versus things like "The audience has reacted very well to me in the past" or "I've prepared thoroughly" or "I have a lot of experience in my field." The following step is to reframe the negative thoughts with more balanced and realistic alternatives like "I've prepared well, and I can handle unexpected questions" or "Not everyone will agree with me, and that's okay." Then consider how these alternative thoughts make you feel.

When we're faced with a hurdle, such as a health issue, we have the chance to examine our thinking and work to diffuse fear by asking ourselves questions like "Do I have the resources around me that will help me meet this challenge? If not, how can I get them? Can I incorporate this news or event into my life without it overwhelming my sense of myself?" Simply by asking ourselves these questions, we're expanding our thinking in a way that minimizes fear and opens us up to problem-solving. CBT helps us gain confidence in our ability to be, in a word, resilient: It shows us that we always have the option to change the way we think; how we process and manage our emotions; and how we'll act in response to a challenge. CBT can help us move through fear.

Barlow advocates for this approach, one that's built around active engagement with one's anticipatory fear. He's done a tremendous amount of research that shows that well-structured and professionally supervised cognitive behavioral therapy helps people with severe or chronic anxiety learn that they can be quite anxious about something . . . and yet still act. The key CBT techniques are exposure therapy, which we've discussed, and cognitive restructuring, which challenges negative thoughts or cognitive distortions such as all-or-nothing thinking, overgeneralization, catastrophizing, or personalization (blaming yourself for things that are outside your control). These approaches do not try to circumvent or avoid the anxiety; instead, they accept that anxiety is a natural aspect of the human experience and that if we learn to work with it—rather than avoid it—we reclaim a vital aspect of our agency. How do we do this? By accepting anxiety as a normal, albeit uncomfortable emotional response. Being willing to challenge our thinking and beliefs around fear is essential for building and maintaining resilience.

I have a patient, a young woman named Emily, who suffered preeclampsia after giving birth to her first child. We controlled her blood pressure through medication, but her fear of having high blood pressure made her literally afraid to do anything after giving birth. Although she had once been an active runner, she was petrified about starting to exercise again. Her life became hard to enjoy because of her health-related anxiety. Together we worked slowly on regulating and monitoring her blood pressure. She also sought treatment with a therapist, who helped her work on her anxiety around this health event. Over the course of a year, we were able to finally get her off blood pressure medication. She now no longer checks her blood pressure multiple times a day as she did before and has gone back to exercising and enjoying life.

Every challenge we face provides an opportunity to learn and grow. We test out new coping mechanisms, problem-solving skills, and emotional-regulation strategies. These skills then become valuable additions to our tool kit, making it easier to navigate future challenges. In essence, each successful experience with adversity strengthens our resilience. This creates a virtuous cycle where resilience begets further resilience, leading to greater personal growth and an improved quality of life.

Speaking of tools, I also conferred with psychologist Jonathan DePierro, PhD, the director of Mount Sinai's Center for Stress, Resilience and Personal Growth, about how we can learn to take action, even in the face of fear. He recommended taking a "stepwise" approach. "It's all about setting small goals and meeting those goals one at a time," DePierro said. "If you've had a heart attack, you may start with just taking a few steps across the room, before walking around the block, then up and down a hill, then perhaps jogging or running—not all in one day but over the course of days and weeks."

Taking small steps can help you both physically and mentally. Any kind of difficult event or challenging circumstances can throw our sense of identity into crisis. For example, it's not uncommon for my patients to have to grapple with incorporating a diagnosis of chronic illness into their concept of themselves. Often, patients experience a sense of shame when they're given a diagnosis. I hear things like "If only I hadn't smoked when I was young." Or "I should have paid more attention to my diet." This kind of self-recrimination, however, only feeds into the negative feelings that can leave us depressed or anxious.

Dr. DePierro shared that he sometimes suggests an exercise in cognitive reframing when a patient's self-image is in danger of being overwhelmed by a diagnosis. He suggests drawing a circle and then writing at the top, *I am a person who* . . . The next task is to allot sections of that circle, or pie, to various aspects of one's identity. For example, the most important role in your life might be as a mother or father, so this would take up a large slice of the pie; or you may realize that more than half of the pie is for your role as a partner and a valued family member; the next significant slice might be your job or profession; then the next might be your hobby or what you love to do with your spare time. When you finally get to where the medical diagnosis fits in, there is usually only a thin slice of the identity pie left. And this is how it should be. When we consciously explore our sense of who we are, in all its many facets, we find that a medical diagnosis just doesn't carry the same weight as the important roles in our lives. Of course, over the course of one's life, our various roles expand, contract, and fluctuate, but this kind of exercise helps us move out of fear and into a self-supporting mindset, which helps us hang on to a more concrete, more realistic sense of who we are.

I don't want to minimize in any way how scary it is to get a serious medical diagnosis; it is scary. But as you practice the Resilience Response, you don't have to stay afraid.

CHAPTER 7

Build Connections

Alone we can do so little; together we can do so much.
—Helen Keller

As a resident, working late nights and in stressful situations with people means you get to know a lot about them in a short time. One of my colleagues I liked a lot, Charles, shared stories of his growing up in a large working-class family. His father, who worked in a machine shop, was gruff and remote. His mother worked part-time at a local pharmacy. Charles was the youngest, and despite his loud and rambunctious household, he later recounted to me how lonely he often felt—despite sharing a bedroom with his two brothers and eating dinner with his family every night. Other kids always told him his family was "fun," and as a child he felt obligated to act as though this were true. But it didn't feel fun to him—he was often teased by his older siblings for preferring books over sports and solitude to a crowd. "I often felt like I was so different from the rest of my family that I must have been adopted or something," he once joked.

Every child in his family was described a certain way: his oldest brother was the "jock," and his oldest sister was "the slob," and so on. Charles was the "smart one," which was both a blessing and a curse. His parents loved that he brought home straight A's, while several of his siblings—especially his brothers—resented him for this. And it made Charles believe he needed to excel at school to be loved, even though doing so also made him feel alienated from those closest to him. He grew up with an unrelenting pressure to perform.

Deep into our residency, that finally caught up with him. One late night he called me and said, "Tara, I don't think I can do it." I could tell by the tone of his voice that something was seriously wrong.

"Do what, Charles?" I found myself getting up out of bed.

"I don't think I can go on. With this work. With any of it." I asked where he was, and I stayed on the phone with him while I got my coat and headed out the door in the direction of his apartment.

Charles and I talked late into the night, and what we talked about was loneliness. I had experienced pretty profound loneliness myself when I was away at school, both as an undergrad and then during medical school, as I found myself thousands of miles from my loving family. I experienced it again, even more profoundly, when I had to extricate myself from the toxic, controlling romantic relationship I mentioned earlier in the book.

Charles and I were different. I had a supportive and close family. I could talk to my parents about anything going on in my life. Charles didn't have that same resource. He often felt he didn't have *anyone* he could turn to. That night, after our conversation, I fell asleep on his couch, mulling over how best I could help him. Over coffee in the morning, I asked Charles if he would ever consider seeing a therapist. I could tell this was a new idea for him, but he agreed to give it a try.

Build Connections

We made some calls and found someone who would see him that day. He started therapy immediately.

Our friendship grew stronger as he shared with me what he was learning about his perfectionism. He was beginning to realize how it kept him at a distance from other people, even as a child. He explained what a relief it was to find out that feeling lonely while growing up in a big family wasn't unusual. He interrogated more of his key beliefs—including that he had to perform to be lovable.

In just a few short months, Charles grew more relaxed and more content. As he began to shed the persona of the overachieving outsider that he'd unconsciously adopted when he was young, he was able to bond more meaningfully with other members of our incredible cohort. He made new, more meaningful friendships. I'm grateful to say, he also deepened the ones he had, including his friendship with me.

Today, Charles is a highly regarded surgeon. He's also happily married and the father of two adorable girls. I felt good that I could help him in a moment of need, as I myself have been the recipient of this kind of care and connection. I have a firsthand understanding of how all it takes is one person seeing you—really seeing you—to make a difference.

So far, we have focused on elements of the Resilience Response that you can tackle, for the most part, by yourself: having a flexible mindset, taking care of your physical health and well-being, facing fears. Now we're going to move into resilience-building steps that require you to engage with others around you, both individuals and the broader communities of which you are a part. The next step that we'll discuss in this chapter, making and sustaining connections with others, is a key ingredient in the Resilience Response.

From the moment we're born, we begin to orient ourselves in the world in relation to the people in our lives. The quality of our earliest relationships, with our parents or our primary caregivers, influences how well we'll relate to others as we age. John Bowlby, the late British psychologist and psychiatrist, was the father of what we today call attachment theory. This is the philosophy that our early needs make us seek emotional bonds from a predictable caregiver, or attachment figure, that we can rely on especially when we feel distress. Perhaps you've heard about different "attachment styles"—for example, secure attachment, anxious-ambivalent attachment, dismissive-avoidant attachment, and fearful-avoidant attachment. These categorizations are derived from work that Bowlby did from the 1950s until his death in 1990, in which he studied children and their parents. He understood that having a safe and respectful bonding experience as an infant—what we now call secure attachment—helps us meet life's challenges with resilience.

To further develop this theory, Bowlby studied children from various backgrounds. One study focused on children who were separated from their caregivers during World War II and found that they suffered from psychological and emotional problems because of this lack of healthy bonding. Without the loving, consistent care of their parents, these children later had difficulty forming healthy and trusting relationships with others. Another study focused on what were then referred to as "illegitimate children," or children who were born to unwed mothers. These children often did not remain with their birth mothers as they grew up, and this lack of stability, Bowlby argued, led to delinquency. In a 1952 report entitled "Maternal Care and Mental Health," Bowlby asserted that damage caused by a lack of meaningful interpersonal attachment early in life can hinder social and emotional development in crucial ways later in life.

I had the enormous benefit of being raised in a supportive and loving family where I felt close to both of my parents. That said, I am also no stranger to the challenges that can come with trying to connect to others

Build Connections

when we feel isolated or alone. A mentor of mine in medical school, Dr. Astrid Heger, helped me come through an incredibly dark period in my life. Dr. Heger, a professor of pediatric medicine, taught in a way that spoke directly to me: She understood that being a good doctor wasn't about identifying an illness or making a diagnosis. That was the obvious, even easy, part of the job. A good doctor, she believed, was a healer. As doctors we could only truly heal people if we invested in the lives of our patients, if we connected to them as human beings, not only in their medical outcomes. In addition to helping me see the personal value of connection, she taught me about the *medical* value of connection.

While I was dealing with that difficult, controlling romantic relationship and was simultaneously afraid I was going to go blind, I heard her give a lecture on helping women extract themselves from abusive situations. Afterward she took a group of female medical students under her wing, inviting us to regular gatherings at her home. With her support and the support of my female classmates, I was able to let go of both fears that gripped me. I could rely on my own strength and that of this supportive community and move forward. I left the controlling romantic relationship soon thereafter. That to build my resilience I could rely on the resilience of others was a powerful discovery. I didn't have to navigate that path alone; others were doing it alongside me, and others had done it before and I could follow their examples. That made me feel less lonely.

I drew upon this power of connection when I started my internship and residency at Brigham and Women's Hospital in Boston—a time of grueling challenges that came with caring for patients as a new doctor. I was scared I would kill someone, worried I would not learn enough, quickly enough, and I was almost always exhausted from the lack of sleep. My first rotation was on the bone-marrow-transplant service, where I took care of possibly the sickest patients one can imagine. These patients are so vulnerable, so precarious, as their entire immune systems are wiped out in preparation for accepting new stem cells, that they are kept in an almost bubble-like protective state. Every precaution is taken to prevent them from getting an infection in those first few weeks. They also look emaciated, hovering on the brink of death. I remember leaving my rotations and crying in the stairwell, overwhelmed from seeing people in this state and hoping I could do right by them. I worried that whatever I could do as a doctor might not be enough.

In those early months I was lucky to meet a few fellow female interns who would quickly become my tribe. I recall meeting them for dinner on one of our rare nights off. I felt utterly spent, and I wondered aloud how I could possibly continue. One by one they lifted me up. I remember my friend Julie saying, "Tara, we got you. And you've got this. We won't let you fall." From that day on until today, they have held to their promise, and I, too, have been able to return it to them in kind. These nine women have become my best friends. We saw each other through the challenge of residency and have since weathered the many ups and downs of life together, including births, deaths, marriages, divorce, and illness. I am forever grateful that my training brought them into my life and showed me the power of connection.

My former medical-school mentor Dr. Heger—Astrid—has also become a beloved friend. She is a true healthcare trailblazer. A USC Keck School of Medicine graduate herself, she was one of the first people to conduct medical research into child exploitation and sexual abuse. She later returned to USC to join the faculty and create a program that would establish a standard of care for both women and children who had been victims of sexual abuse, at a time when these public-health issues were barely discussed. Heger's passion led her to create the Center for the Vul-

Build Connections

nerable Child in 1984, the first medically based child advocacy program in the world. She understood that treating the medical issues these children faced was only the first step. She knew that, for these young people to overcome the trauma they had experienced, they would need to be provided with food, clothing, shelter, medical services, mental health services—and more. She has been devoted to this work ever since.

Healing for these children entails, as Heger puts it, "restoring their personal essence." This means going the extra mile and helping a girl shuttling from one foster home to another to buy a prom dress, or working the phones until Heger finds a plastic surgeon who will repair a battered child's face, or getting a car fixed so one of her teenage patients can make it to their therapy appointment. Connecting these children to others who can help and support them as they recover is the key.

Nearly fifty years after her career began, Dr. Heger is still working as hard as ever, now as the executive director of the Violence Intervention Program (VIP), which serves over twenty thousand children in need a year. I still remember the words from one of her early lectures: "You have to make medicine personal because it is personal." She showed me the power of connection in a clinical setting, and it has been such a guiding principle for me. That's why I keep talking about how we must truly get to know our patients to help them heal. If healing is about restoring and maintaining quality of daily life, just putting a stent in someone's heart won't do it. You must understand what their daily life is all about. Building connection with a patient is how. That begins with doctors taking the time to ask their patients who they are and whom they are striving to become, and patients sharing.

The examples of Charles and Dr. Heger and of me finding my tribe of women during my residency all underscore the importance of connection as we face challenges in our lives. It informs how I live and how I practice. But I also want to dive into the consequences—physically, emotionally, and spiritually—of what happens when we don't have enough connection.

How Loneliness Affects Our Minds and Bodies

But before we go further, let's get clearer on what we mean, medically speaking, when we talk about loneliness. Loneliness is a significant psychosocial stressor, one with measurable physical and psychological consequences. A subjective feeling of distress, it is nevertheless linked to very concrete health risks.

Psychologically speaking, we've come to understand that loneliness is the gap between the social connections you have, and the ones you would like to have. This disconnection can then lead to feelings of isolation even when in the presence of others. As comedian Robin Williams said, "I used to think the worst thing in life was to end up all alone. It's not. The worst thing in life is to end up with people who make you feel all alone." That's exactly what Charles felt as a child, too.

You can be in a crowd and feel lonely. And you can be alone and feel lonely, too. But Louise Hawkley, a senior research scientist at the National Opinion Research Center (NORC) at the University of Chicago, is careful to point out that loneliness and being alone are not at all the same. Being alone, she reminds us, is an objective state and often promotes health by giving the individual, spending time in solitude by choice, the chance to rest and rejuvenate. Feeling lonely, in contrast, is a subjective state and can be experienced, as I've mentioned, even while we are with others.

The loneliness expert and pioneer in social neuroscience, the late John Cacioppo, was one of the first to identify that our innate need to connect with others is essential for optimal health and well-being. Hawkley described loneliness as a subjective state; Cacioppo viewed loneliness as a problem of perception; he emphasized that loneliness is not determined by the objective number of social connections a person has, but rather by their subjective experience of those connections. Someone might have many social contacts, but if they feel those relationships lack depth, meaning, or emotional connection, they can still experience profound loneliness. On the other hand, someone with fewer social contacts might not feel lonely if they perceive their existing relationships as satisfying. Cacioppo also focused on "perceived social isolation" in his work, the feeling of being disconnected or excluded, even if objectively one is not. The perceptions of loneliness and social isolation are influenced by many factors, including one's history, personality, mindset, socioeconomic forces, and so much more. And regardless of what influences this perception, it has a powerful influence on our biological health.

Loneliness can contribute to myriad physical and mental-health issues: aggressive behaviors, social anxiety, cognitive decline and the progression of Alzheimer's disease, recurrent stroke, obesity, elevated blood pressure, sleep issues, and suppressed immunity, among others. In a coauthored review published in the *Annals of the New York Academy of Sciences*, Hawkley and Cacioppo detailed how loneliness contributes to increased activation of the hypothalamic-pituitary-adrenal (HPA) axis, the body's primary stress-response system, leading to decreased inflammatory control and problems with immunity and sleep—all of which increased mortality rates in older adults. It turns out that loneliness can, in fact, kill.

Here's how and why loneliness can have such profound effects on the physical body and the brain.

First, the body senses what it interprets as a threat, even though in reality the threat is only imagined. Cacioppo's work often drew from an evolutionary perspective to explain this. He theorized that loneliness evolved as a warning signal, alerting individuals to potential threats to their survival. In ancestral environments, we relied on one another for most things, and social isolation could have been a death sentence. Nowadays, the perception of isolation still triggers a response, even if the actual threat is not immediate or physical.

Persistent loneliness, then, is a potent stressor, setting in motion a complex cascade of physiological and neurological changes that profoundly impact both the body and the brain. Think of your genes as switches that control what your cells do. When you're lonely, these switches start flipping in a specific pattern. Scientists call this pattern the conserved transcriptional response to adversity, or CTRA. The brain produces corticotropin-releasing hormone (CRH) in response to the alarm—a hormone that kicks off a process whereby our heart rate goes up, our senses become heightened, our digestive and reproductive systems slow down, and our circadian rhythm, hunger, and thirst all get thrown out of whack. But when our loneliness doesn't dissipate, we can't get back to baseline.

In the body, our immune function is impaired, inflammation increases, and we are at increased risk of cardiovascular problems. Part of this stems from the disruption of the delicate balance of the body's HPA axis, our primary stress-response system, as I mentioned earlier in this book. This triggers sustained cortisol release, which affects various systems. It can lead to weakened immune response partly because it triggers us to over-release norepinephrine, which can temporarily suppress some of the body's immune functions. A chronic inflammatory response can also weaken the body's overall ability to respond to new infections.

As mentioned, loneliness also takes a toll on the cardiovascular system. It does so because it directly affects our sympathetic nervous system, the part responsible for the fight, flight, or freeze response. When activated, it releases hormones such as adrenaline, which increases our heart rate and causes blood pressure to rise. In lonely individuals, this system is constantly revved up, leading to chronically elevated heart rate and blood pressure. Over time, this sustained stress puts extra wear and tear on the heart, increasing the risk of heart disease. As we've seen, loneliness triggers inflammation throughout the body—and this includes the heart and blood vessels. Inflammation damages the delicate lining of the arteries, making them more prone to plaque buildup. This narrowing of the arteries restricts blood flow to the heart or brain, and when the flow is severely reduced or blocked, it can lead to a heart attack or stroke. Adding to the problem, loneliness can also affect the way blood vessels respond to stress. Normally, your blood vessels should be able to relax and widen when needed, allowing for increased blood flow. But in lonely individuals these vessels can become less flexible, a condition known as endothelial dysfunction. This reduced flexibility makes it harder for your heart to get the oxygen-rich blood it needs, especially when the body is being taxed by physical exertion or psychological stress.

The brain is affected by loneliness, too, in both its structure and function, particularly in regions we use for social cognition, emotion regulation, and executive function. The chronic stress and inflammation brought about by loneliness can cause neuronal damage and reduce our neuroplasticity, affecting our normal levels of neurotransmitters and the size and function of the prefrontal cortex, amygdala, and hippocampus. Loneliness can also contribute to poor sleep quality and insomnia. This and several of the other issues mentioned combined can lead to cognitive issues including impaired memory and attention, and problems with executive function.

Stress caused by the fight, flight, or freeze response takes a physical toll, and an emotional one. Think of loneliness as a magnifying glass, making everything feel much bigger and more intense than it really is. If you're suffering from loneliness, you might find yourself overreacting to things that wouldn't normally bother you, such as a friend canceling plans at the last minute. Instead of brushing it off or feeling slightly hurt or bothered, you might feel that they don't care about you at all, even if they have a perfectly good reason for not showing up. Or, if someone at work makes a slightly critical comment about something you've done, you might take it as a personal attack, even if it was meant to be constructive. You might also become highly attuned to any sign of rejection. If you see a group of people laughing and talking without you, you might automatically assume they're talking about you, even if they're complete strangers you're walking by in the park. A casual, slightly offhand remark can send you spiraling into feelings of intense sadness or anger.

These magnified and distorted perceptions can then lead to social withdrawal. Being overly worried about being hurt or rejected, you might start avoiding social situations altogether. You stop calling friends or your family because you're afraid of being a burden or saying the wrong thing. You might even avoid going to the grocery store or other public places because you're worried about running into people and how they will behave and how you will respond.

This is where the negative feedback of loneliness locks in. Because you're avoiding people, you don't experience any *positive* social interactions, which then makes you feel even more lonely. This loneliness then makes you more sensitive to rejection, which makes you likely to close yourself off further. Your brain is trying to protect you from getting hurt, but it's actually making things worse, misinterpreting benign input as a potential threat. This vicious cycle that loneliness sets in motion takes a real toll on our physical and mental health.

Build Connections

As a healthcare provider, I worry about the toll that the chronic stress of loneliness takes on our mental and biological resilience, making us even more vulnerable to the eventual—yet preventable—onset of a whole host of health and wellness problems. And my worry is not unfounded: Studies show that loneliness is estimated to be alarmingly correlated with a 32 percent increase in the onset of diabetes, a 29 percent increase in the onset of cardiovascular diseases, and a staggering increase of 50 percent in cognitive impairments such as dementia. And, according to the National Institute on Aging, loneliness and social isolation may shave up to fifteen years off the average American's life. That's a shocking 20 percent drop in the expected lifespan of seventy-five years. According to this report, the serious health risks associated with being lonely or isolated, including the toll it takes on our longevity, are more damaging than everything from environmental stressors such as air pollution, being obese, or being sedentary. Most shocking is the evidence that loneliness is more harmful to our health than having six alcoholic drinks a day or smoking fifteen cigarettes a day. In other words, again, loneliness can be lethal.

How can we break through?

To state the obvious, loneliness is not a problem that can be solved by oneself alone. And more and more of us, unfortunately, are experiencing loneliness, and having trouble knowing where to turn. In the spring of 2023 US Surgeon General Vivek Murthy (who is also a longtime friend, fellow Floridian, and child of Indian immigrants, and who was once my resident while I was an intern at Brigham and Women's Hospital) took the unprecedented step of issuing an advisory statement calling out loneliness as a national public-health crisis. Not only did he name it a crisis, he made it clear that we needed to address it immediately and simultaneously announced steps and policies to help do so. When I interviewed Vivek in 2021, he shared two particularly poignant stories with me about his own experiences with loneliness. One was from his childhood, when, he said, "I sometimes faked having a stomachache—I haven't really told my parents about that to this day. I didn't want to go to school because I was scared about being alone again on the playground or in the cafeteria." And he also felt a deep loneliness later, even at the height of his professional accomplishments: "After I left the position of surgeon general [the] last time, I went through a long period of feeling unmoored, disconnected from community—unsure what my purpose was. And that was a very lonely time."

In the report entitled *Our Epidemic of Loneliness and Isolation*, Murthy and his multidisciplinary advisory board compiled longitudinal studies and a vast body of research and data from a broad cross section of disciplines, including psychology, sociology, economics, neuroscience, cardiology, and public health, among others. These kinds of studies illuminate the sheer scale of the problem. A significant portion of the US population experiences loneliness. It affects people of all ages, but findings showed that young adults and older adults are especially vulnerable. Data from the National Poll on Healthy Aging, published in *JAMA*, found that in 2024 one-third of older adults (ages fifty to eighty) reported feeling lonely some of the time or often in the previous year. During and since the pandemic, we also saw an uptick in loneliness among young people. Alarmingly, a report by healthcare company Cigna entitled "The Loneliness Epidemic Persists: A Post-Pandemic Look at the State of Loneliness Among U.S. Adults" cites that an astounding 79 percent of adults aged eighteen to twenty-four report feeling lonely compared to 41 percent of seniors aged sixty-six and older.

Build Connections

As many of us learned firsthand during the pandemic, interacting through a screen is not the same as meeting in person to adequately get our social needs met. As multiple studies have shown, excessive screen time is associated with a range of negative mental-health outcomes such as low emotional stability and greater risk for depression or anxiety. But more and more of us are spending time on our phones or devices rather than being with one another in person. According to a March 2024 Allconnect report, the average screen time for American adults has increased by 60 percent since the outbreak of COVID. Simultaneously, in-person interaction has gone down. In a February 2023 study, researchers tracked smartphone usage in 325 Android-phone users over six days and found that the more people used their smartphones, the less social connectedness they experienced, which led them to use their smartphones more.

And this phenomenon isn't just borne out in the data—I'm sure we all have anecdotal evidence that backs it up. Have you ever absentmindedly hopped onto Facebook to check what your friends are up to only to find that it seems every family you know is off on a seemingly delightful vacation while you're stuck at home, burned-out from work, and struggling to muster any enthusiasm for your daily routine? I know I have, and I've learned to catch myself when I feel my mood begin to sink. But it's harder for young people to resist the addictive lure of logging on to catch a glimpse of the fabulous life of the latest influencer—even when that life is highly curated and digitally enhanced. Being pulled into the vortex can do a number on anyone's sense of self-esteem—but even more so for younger people. They must navigate a highly competitive digital world where false representation is rampant and where bullying and unfiltered criticism are the norm.

The Healing Power of Resilience

And spending too much time online, for all of us, but especially the young, may lead to, or enhance, alienation . . . and loneliness, along with all the chronic stress that brings.

Another critical finding was the economic impact of loneliness. Social isolation means increased healthcare costs, reduced productivity, and diminished civic engagement. Loneliness isn't just a personal problem; it's a societal issue with far-reaching consequences.

So what can we do about this epidemic of loneliness?

The surgeon general's report addressed the importance of changing how we conceive of loneliness and what we should do about it, citing six "pillars" to advance social connection:

Strengthen social infrastructure in local communities
Enact pro-connection public policies
Mobilize the health sector
Reform digital environments
Deepen our knowledge
Cultivate a culture of connection

The report talks about developing programs that help people engage in their communities and prioritize their social health at the local, state, and national level, and within a diverse set of industries. It's an important step toward addressing the loneliness epidemic.

But there is other research on this topic. One of my favorites is one of the longest ongoing health studies ever conducted. It focuses on what turns out to be the key antidote to loneliness. The study, originally known as the Grant Study of Adult Development, began during the Great Depression in 1938. W. T. Grant, a department store magnate, gave Harvard sixty thousand dollars to track two groups of men throughout life to see if the predictors of healthy aging could be identified. One group was made up of Harvard sophomores, the other of disadvantaged youth from Boston's poorest neighborhoods. Today, under the guidance of the fourth director of the study, Robert Waldinger, data has been gathered on more than two thousand subjects spanning three generations. This study has shown that such things as financial wealth, social prestige, or other markers we typically associate with success are not what make people happy and keep them healthy; warm relationships are.

In a Ted Talk viewed by more than forty-six million people, Waldinger outlines how the seventy-five years of data gathered by Harvard, when examined along with other overlapping studies, shows clearly that the number one predictor of health and longevity is how satisfied we are in our personal relationships. It's about having that one person we know we can call in the middle of the night, when we're distressed or in trouble or we simply need to connect. It's also about our relationships with our colleagues, our neighbors, the people we see every week at the gym, and even the strangers we smile at on the street. These so-called warm connections help alleviate the stress of loneliness. So what are they, how can we develop them, and what else can we do to fight back against loneliness when we experience it?

Tools to Fight Loneliness

If we are stuck in a cycle of loneliness, it can be difficult to reach out and ask for help. Or to let those around us know that we need them. But there are small steps we can take toward connection, especially toward building the warm connections mentioned above that can help us break out of the loneliness spiral. Scientifically speaking, warm connections are social interactions that activate specific neurobiological pathways, leading to measurable physiological and psychological changes. There are a few, but I'll talk about two I find fascinating. First, such interactions spur the release of oxytocin, a neuropeptide that plays a pivotal role in social bonding and stress reduction. Second, warm connections influence the autonomic nervous system, helping us switch from sympathetic dominance (characterized by fight, flight, or freeze responses) to parasympathetic activation (rest-and-digest mode), which lowers our heart rate, blood pressure, and cortisol levels. Brain regions associated with reward and positive reinforcement activate the release of dopamine and other neurotransmitters that enhance feelings of pleasure and well-being. Essentially, warm connections represent a complex interplay of brain and hormonal mechanisms that promote social attachment, emotional regulation, and overall well-being.

That means that breaking out of loneliness requires a degree of retraining your brain, which, thanks to neuroplasticity, is possible at any age. It helps to first show some self-compassion. Acknowledge that loneliness isn't a personal failing; it's a common human experience. Try to talk to yourself internally with the same kindness and understanding you'd offer a friend. When negative thoughts creep in, such as "No one likes me," look for evidence to challenge this thought. Our brains have a negativity bias, meaning we tend to focus on the negative (a great survival technique when we were living subsistence lifestyles, but not so much anymore), so you have to actively reframe your thoughts. Mindfulness techniques can help with this. Even a few minutes of daily meditation can help you become more aware of your thoughts and feelings without judgment, reducing the power of those negative thought patterns.

Next, focus on building those warm connections. This isn't about having a huge social circle; it's about quality over quantity. The phrase *find, remind, and bind* can be a great shorthand way to help us think about how we can break out of our feelings of isolation. This simple yet powerful framework helps us take a mindful approach to connecting with others. The *find* step involves actively seeking out and noticing the good things that others do. Sounds easy, and it can be if you're in the right frame of mind—being present and observant. If you are out of practice, start small. Take your time. The more you do this, the more small acts of kindness you will see.

The *bind* step is about articulating your appreciation sincerely and specifically, explaining why someone's actions or qualities are meaningful to you—helping them to feel validated and seen. Choose one thing you've observed to share with someone else. For example, you could share with a colleague, "I find that you always bring a positive attitude to our meetings, even when things are challenging." The *remind* step is about reinforcing the positive connection by reminding the other person of their value and the impact they have on your life. It's an expression of appreciation over time, not just a onetime occurrence. For example, by saying something like "I'm reminded when we talk how much I appreciate your friendship and how your support has helped me through this latest challenge." The more you do this, the easier it becomes. If you encounter a setback—for instance, someone responds to you in a less than positive manner, or you find yourself feeling awkward—that's okay. You can always go back to collecting positives you observe before you again feel ready to try to share something aloud.

Try to be patient and persistent. Building meaningful connections takes time and effort and, again, is a form of cognitive retraining. Just like exercise, the rewards don't come immediately. Every interaction is a new opportunity to practice and refine your social skills. Celebrate small victories and acknowledge your progress.

Physical touch is another way to combat feelings of loneliness and bring stress down. Physical sensations such as hugging, cuddling, and hand-holding stimulate the release of oxytocin. Oxytocin, which we'll revisit later, is often referred to as the bonding hormone or love hormone. It plays a crucial role in social bonding, promoting feelings of trust and connection, and, you guessed it, in reducing stress. On the flip side, chronic stress and resulting high cortisol levels can interfere with oxytocin signaling by reducing oxytocin receptor sensitivity, thus interfering with the ability of oxytocin to exert its calming effects. Under conditions of extreme stress, cortisol may directly suppress oxytocin production, creating a negative feedback loop that leads to HPA-axis dysregulation. Conversely, when we experience physical touch, our brain releases the chemical signals that can correct the physiological dysregulation caused by the stress and return us to equilibrium.

But even if we know that relationships, especially ones that include physical touch, are the key out of despair, finding lasting and meaningful connection is not always so simple. Dan Siegel, a professor of psychiatry at the UCLA School of Medicine and the cofounding director of the Mindful Awareness Research Center at UCLA, specializes in the field of interpersonal neurobiology. This relatively new and interdisciplinary field explores the intricate connections between the brain, the mind, and relationships, looking to understand how our interactions with others shape our neural development and mental processes, and conversely, how our brains influence our relationships. Building on Bowlby's research, Siegel identified what he calls the Four S's of healthy early attachment, which are the four basic experiences he posits children need to develop optimally, to reach their full potential and thrive in all aspects of life. The Four S's are feeling seen, being safe, being soothed, and feeling secure.

Let's unpack them one by one. When we're "seen" by others, this is shorthand for the feeling of being valued for our authentic selves: separate, unique, and worthy of deep love and respect.

Build Connections

When we feel safe with another, it means that person cares about our welfare and our well-being and won't intentionally harm us. Being soothed means that we'll have people around to comfort us when we're sad, stressed, or overcome emotionally. When we feel secure—namely, when we don't feel the need to modulate who we are to receive validation—we can engage with the world with confidence and a sense of ease. We can take on challenges, make mistakes without collapsing, and grow our resilience.

For some of us, a lack of healthy attachment when we're young, as Bowlby first explained, can set us up for trouble later in life. But it's never too late to build healthy attachments and to overcome the harmful toll loneliness takes on us, body, mind, and spirit.

I would argue that the presence of the Four S's is the foundation for great relationships throughout our life. Seek out these connections. This can be with a friend, a family member, or a stranger. It doesn't even necessarily have to be a big heart-to-heart conversation to have an impact, as Waldinger's research shows. Though one interaction will not solve loneliness permanently, any in-person social interaction can be a mood booster. A study done in the middle of the COVID pandemic, when face-to-face contact proved harder to come by, showed that daily face-to-face contact was particularly beneficial in mitigating depression.

We've all heard stories about someone who has stood in line for a coffee, and when it's their turn at the counter, the barista tells them that the person in front of them (who is already out the door) has paid for their drink. I have witnessed my mom perform small acts of kindness over and over—paying for someone's groceries, helping someone who has tripped and needs a hand, going out of her way to hold the door for an elderly person; we can all do such things any time any day. Any gesture of generosity like this can create enough of a spark of good feeling in us that it can, even ever so slightly, shift our mood and our mindset and momentarily lift us out of loneliness. This is because for that one, unexpected moment, we were *seen*. (And, it's worth noting, we only ever saw the back of the person who had acknowledged us!) When we stepped up to order, and the barista looked us in the eye and said, in effect, this is a gift for you, we became connected to the rest of humanity in a profoundly meaningful, even loving, way.

I try to remember that these types of interactions go both ways. You may be lonely, even depressed, but if you can muster the will to be the one to buy a bagel for a stranger or to hold a door, the beneficial effects will be the same: Your willingness to acknowledge another person will have the same positive effect on your mood as if you were the one acknowledged. It will give you just enough of a social and emotional bump to lift you out of your loneliness, however briefly. These encounters remind us that we are valuable members of humanity.

Of course, even many thirty-second exchanges with strangers won't fortify you enough to assuage loneliness. You will have to learn to share yourself with others in more meaningful and challenging ways, including identifying and being willing to share your feelings, openly and honestly, with people who truly care about you. To do that, you must do the hard work of being open and honest with yourself.

In his bestselling book, *Together: The Healing Power of Human Connection in a Sometimes Lonely World*, Surgeon General Vivek Murthy, MD, who obviously takes loneliness seriously as evidenced by the report we explored earlier, writes about our need to "befriend" ourselves to do the work to combat our loneliness. If we didn't grow up with the kind of early attachment or attention that nourishes and fertilizes within us a strong and positive sense of self, then this "befriending" can be quite challenging.

Build Connections

One particularly destructive inner voice that loneliness may bring is the voice of comparison, where we compare how we're feeling with what we're seeing in the outside world, when we feel like we are worse off than those around us, regardless of whether that is true. Back in my lowest moment of medical school, it was particularly challenging to look around and see my peers, who appeared to be thriving. I had no idea what they thought or felt, but I assumed they were much better off than I. I found myself feeling isolated.

What I was feeling back then can be summed up by the saying "compare and despair." I love that saying. When we're feeling low and lonely, and we compare ourselves to others, we tend to assume that their internal reality is more positive than ours. But it's just an assumption. To effectively counteract the stress of loneliness, you must be willing to meet yourself where you are and accept your current loneliness, isolation, or alienation with openheartedness and genuine curiosity. At those gatherings in medical school, Astrid helped me think differently about what I was feeling, and what I assumed my peers were feeling. She helped me let my guard down about what was going on in my personal life and how it was affecting my sense of self-worth. Once I could be open and honest with myself, I could be open and honest with my peers and connect with them.

Another distinct memory from my residency reminds me to be open and honest with myself and my peers. I had to lead a weekly clinic as part of training in how to care for outpatients. My session was on Thursday afternoons from one to five, when I would see as many patients as I could. Not only was I in training and so wanted to be doubly sure about every exam I did and every bit of advice I gave, but I am also a bit of a perfectionist, so I didn't exactly zip through these evaluations. I read every note from prior doctors, carefully reviewed labs, consulted any imaging, and discussed everything these patients saw as important.

The Healing Power of Resilience

Unsurprisingly, it took me a long time to finish with each patient. I never finished before 6:00 p.m. I felt as if I were a failure. All of my peers seemed able to see all of their patients in the allotted time. How would I ever have a full practice as a doctor if I couldn't efficiently and properly manage even six patients? I felt a bit despondent.

Each of us had an attending internal primary-care physician as a mentor. I was assigned to Dr. James Winshall. He was an incredible physician, a husband, a father of three. One night as I was walking out late again, I saw Jamie in his office. He called out to me to stop in for a moment. When he complimented me on a job well done that day, I had to fight back tears. He told me to sit down and asked what was wrong. I remember telling him I felt I was letting him down and that I must have been the worst intern he had mentored. He gently advised me to stop being so hard on myself and told me that being as kind with myself as I was to my patients would help me a lot. I thanked him and went home, still feeling gloomy.

I later opened my email, and there was a message from Jamie: "I'm worried that you think you are not doing a good job. Nothing could be further from the truth. You have everything it takes to be a great doctor, even if you will always finish later than everyone else. Stay away from the negative thoughts. Let's work together to make this a fun and productive year." Those few lines made me feel connected to Jamie.

It didn't matter how many more patients my peers were able to see in the same amount of time. I was doing my best, and it was more than good enough. Jamie saw in me what I could not see in myself. He helped me find my resilience in his simple act of kindness.

Just a few days later while riding his motorized scooter home one night, Jamie was struck by a tractor trailer and killed. His death was

Build Connections

a tragedy on so many levels. For me, it was another reminder of how meaningful connections are. I have saved his email all these years, and sometimes now after a day of seeing twenty patients in my cardiology practice, I smile and think of how far I have come, still thorough but more efficient. And I smile at how proud Jamie would be of his mentee.

Once you know how to start, there are many ways of connecting meaningfully with others. The good news is we have unlimited opportunities to do so each and every day—but we do have to act to make these connections. It's worth it, even if it feels awkward or scary. If one-on-one connections feel too intimidating a place to begin, seek out connection in a group activity or gathering. A book group. A hiking or walking or bridge club. A volunteer group where you can tackle a cause with others who care about it. Or a support group that helps you address an issue you'd like to work on or that you have recovered from. I'll put in a plug here for one of my favorites: The Go Red for Women initiative, begun by the American Heart Association in 2004, helps raise awareness about cardiovascular disease—the leading cause of death in women—and how to combat and live with it. The initiative focuses on educating women about their risk factors, encouraging healthy lifestyle choices, and advocating for greater research and resources dedicated to women's heart health. In local chapters women can connect with one another, share their experiences, and find encouragement and support for behavioral changes such as eating healthier and being more physically active. Go Red for Women also hosts events, online communities, and educational programs where women are encouraged to share their stories. This sense of connection with others who have gone through similar challenges helps combat feelings of isolation and also equips women with medical knowledge and a sense of agency that helps them build resilience.

The Healing Power of Resilience

Connections are crucial to your health, both because they work to lessen chronic stress and can help anchor you when you're faced with a health challenge. You should feel you have someone around to support you through as you face it. When I spoke with Dr. Jonathan DePierro, professor of psychiatry at the Icahn School of Medicine at Mount Sinai, about how we can better help our patients find the support they need when they're faced with a health crisis, he recommended that we encourage patients to reach out to their support network before they undergo a surgery or major medical procedure. By alerting those we're close to that we are going to need help, we give them a chance to rally around us.

I've spoken at length in this chapter about places to make new connections, but don't overlook current and past connections—you might be surprised who will show up when you ask for help. When one of my patients, Edward, let people around him know that he was going in for heart surgery, he was surprised when not one, not two, but three separate friends offered to take the day off work and accompany him to and from the hospital. His sister, who lives in another state, took it upon herself to reach out to his best friend and get a list of Edward's contacts so she could set up a schedule for people to deliver food, walk his dog, or just come and visit. Not only did this help alleviate Edward's fear around his upcoming bypass surgery, but it also made him realize how cherished he is by his community. Edward sailed through his surgery, and thanks in no small part to the many warm relationships supporting him through his recovery, it was swift and complication-free. He responded resiliently to this health challenge. When he came to me for a follow-up visit six months later, he told me that he'd begun dating a woman who lived in his neighborhood but whom he hadn't ever spoken to before he needed help. "We used to wave at each other if we saw each

Build Connections

other, but she brought over a delicious home-cooked meal, and when I asked her if she wanted to stay and share it with me, she said yes." He smiled and shook his head. "We've been together ever since."

Being a patient is often a new and vulnerable role for us to take on, and this is, perhaps, the time when tapping into our social support system is most important. DePierro reminded me that it's perfectly all right for me, as a doctor, to remind my patients that "as the Beatles say, we all 'get by with a little help from our friends.'" New or old. And knowing that the research is out there to back me up on it helps.

CHAPTER 8

Seek Out Love

As we contemplate how to build resilience, especially for the prevention or treatment of chronic disease, I can't help but think that it all comes down to love.

A therapist of mine once asked me to do this exercise. He told me to imagine I was blind and was suddenly granted the gift of being able to see, but only for a few minutes before losing my sight again.

He asked, "What would you want to see in those few minutes?"

It took me only a second to answer. I said simply, "I would want to see the faces of David, Siena, and Layla," my husband and my two daughters.

In that moment I was flooded with an overpowering sense of gratitude. I vowed that I would do my best to never take my loved ones for granted. I know how incredibly blessed I am to be able to walk through life with people I adore and who adore me—even when I make mistakes. Even when I hurt them. Even when I make decisions they might disagree with. Having this kind of support has fueled my resilience throughout my life, and I know it will carry me to the end.

The therapist looked at me and said, "Tara, you are so blessed; you literally have everything you want right in front of you every day. You just have to keep your eyes open."

Defining love is a notoriously complex task, one that's been tackled by poets, philosophers, scientists, teenagers, and everyone in between for millennia. Love encompasses a wide spectrum of emotions and experiences, but here's my best attempt to break it down to its key elements and differentiate it from simply seeking connections or support—an important distinction when we consider it as part of a Resilience Response.

Love, at its core, is a profound emotional bond characterized by a strong sense of fondness, tenderness, and concern. While love can exist as a feeling within an individual and be directed toward another, or toward the world or humanity (as, for instance, in a religious sense), it is most often understood as a reciprocal experience. Between individuals, love can manifest in various forms, including romantic, familial, and platonic. In all cases where another person is in a loving relationship, it means accepting someone for who they are, flaws and all. It entails understanding their perspectives, needs, and desires and often creates a sense of shared identity and belonging, a feeling of "we" or "us."

Love is a deeper, more enduring, and more emotionally charged bond than simply feeling connected to another. Love is a unique combination of intimacy, commitment, and emotional investment—and a willingness to sacrifice, if needed, something of oneself for the benefit of the other.

Giving love to and receiving it from others, I believe, contributes enormously to our ability to develop or maintain an optimistic or hopeful outlook on the future, even in the midst of enormous hardship, and to our feeling of purpose—all elements of a Resilience Response.

In my practice I get to witness firsthand again and again the relationship between love and resilience. For instance, with Gus, one of my longtime patients.

Seek Out Love

After he suffered a severe stroke, Gus almost became a different man. Before the incident, Gus was pretty gruff and seemed to enjoy acting as though he were truly pissed off with the world. In the immediate aftermath of the stroke, this practiced air of disdain became more pronounced. He was a proud man, and at seventy-five years old, and up until the minute of the stroke—which he had in his office—he was working full-time as a senior litigator at a tony midtown law firm. The stroke forced Gus to take a medical leave of absence while he underwent rehabilitation. This reminder of his body's inherent limitations was a blow to his image of himself as a tough guy. He could no longer hide out behind his Teflon facade.

In my twenty-plus years as a doctor, I have found that when people are used to doing everything for themselves, the need to rely on someone else to walk, to go to the bathroom, to get in and out of bed, can feel even worse than whatever medical issues they might be recovering from. This loss of independence can add insult to injury when we are already being forced to come to grips with our body's inherent limitations as the result of a medical condition. The double psychological impact can be substantial, as for many people independence is deeply intertwined with their personal identity. This loss of agency can lead to feelings of helplessness and frustration and can be particularly challenging for some. Studies of individuals facing chronic illnesses or disabilities have shown a strong correlation between perceived loss of control and increased levels of anxiety, depression, and other mental health issues.

What particularly rankled Gus as he recovered was when his grandchildren, who were young teens, would visit him but just "mumble and stare at their phones." But after a couple of months, his attitude toward them began to change. He told me about his grandson, a "fine" baseball player, and his granddaughter, who wanted to grow up to be a chef, like

The Healing Power of Resilience

"Ina!" "Ina who?" Gus would say. "Ina Garten!" she'd reply. He seemed to marvel at how witty, bright, and active these kids were—as though they had been strangers to him and he was meeting them for the first time. When he was finally out of rehab and came to my office, he took a call from his grandson, who wanted to fill Gus in on his latest game. While they spoke, I watched Gus light up. He was clearly delighted by these smart, interesting young people who, he joked, "just happen to be in my life and want to know me. . . . Can you believe it?"

It struck me hard how Gus was only able to connect at a deeper level—a loving level—with his grandchildren when he was at his most vulnerable. Life had knocked him down, and to get back up, he found a way to allow himself to love and be loved, even by his "know-nothing" grandkids. When I cleared Gus to return to work, he told me that he was going to move into an emeritus role at his firm, in which he could mentor young attorneys. This, he told me somewhat sheepishly, would be a part-time role.

"What will you do with the rest of your time?" I asked, knowing he prided himself on being the toughest and hardest-working attorney at his firm, if not in the city.

"I'm not entirely sure yet," he said thoughtfully, "but you know I have some baseball games to catch, and I might take someone for some cooking classes." As he said this, he winked at me. I knew then that he was just fine. In fact, he was better than ever.

This is the reason I (mostly) don't worry about patients such as Gus who have loving family surrounding them. I worry about patients who are isolated or lacking in social support, or whose networks are more fragile and will be significantly impacted if the patient becomes less independent.

A meta-analysis conducted by Julianne Holt-Lunstad, an expert on social connection and health, found a strong association between social isolation and loneliness and increased mortality risk. As she puts it succinctly, "We need to prioritize our social relationships like our life depends on it, because it does." Given that dealing with or recovering from a medical condition can lead to an accompanying decline in independence, I am concerned about patients who are already lacking social connection. On the contrary, when I give a patient a tough diagnosis and know that they are surrounded by spouses or children or dear close friends, I feel confident that this person will ultimately be okay. Their support system assures me that they're not alone on their journey, that they are buttressed by the kind of love they'll need to meet whatever challenges they may face.

How Love Affects Our Brains and Bodies

Quite simply, I believe that love is the reason we are alive. Giving and receiving love is the wellspring of meaning and satisfaction for us as a species—the only species that has been given the gift of intelligence and consciousness in this unique combination. I do believe that other species experience their own versions and manifestations of love—this is a truly fascinating topic but is too far afield to focus on here.

Instead, let's dig a bit deeper into what love means for our physical health, our overall well-being, and our ability to develop a Resilience Response.

We have already talked about how important acceptance can be in recovering from a medical incident or wrestling with a difficult diagnosis. Acceptance requires that we see people (including ourselves!) in their entirety. This unconditional, some might call it radical, acceptance makes room for us to love ourselves and others. Psychologist, author, and spiritual teacher Tara Brach talks about radical acceptance first as a way to embrace all aspects of ourselves including our imperfections, vulnerabilities, and painful emotions—and then extending that unconditional acceptance to another person, flaws and all.

Love requires moving beyond acceptance to compassion. We can see and acknowledge the suffering that is inherent in life, feel an emotional response to the suffering of others, and respond in a way that we hope can alleviate that suffering. The Dalai Lama says, "Genuine compassion must have both wisdom and loving kindness. That is to say, one must understand the nature of the suffering from which we wish to free others (this is wisdom), and one must experience deep intimacy and empathy with other sentient beings (this is loving kindness)."

For me, compassion is also essential to my practice of medicine. For doctors and nurses, a commitment to relieving the suffering of others is a part of our everyday lives. Cleaning port lines and feeding tubes. Administering painkillers. Discussing prognoses with patients. Offering support to family members when we make difficult diagnoses or at the moment of loss. These are daily tasks for millions of healthcare providers. The American Medical Association's Principles of Medical Ethics states in the very first line that medical services should be rendered with "compassion and respect for human dignity." Even more interesting, studies have shown that compassionate care—the kinds of acts I described above, and more—is associated with better patient outcomes, including reduced anxiety, improved adherence to treatment plans, faster recovery times—and on the caregiver side, a reduction in medical errors.

Research suggests that our brains are naturally wired for helping others. Doing so activates reward centers in the brain, inciting feelings similar to those we experience when eating or enjoying pleasurable activities. This suggests that generosity is biologically beneficial, since we are more likely to repeat behaviors that feel good. For example, one study found that parts of the brain involved in the mesolimbic reward system, the area activated by such stimuli as sex, drugs, food, and receiving money, are also engaged when people make charitable donations. Another study showed that participants' brains lit up in reward-processing areas even when they were forced to give to others—and the level of activity was even higher when they gave voluntarily. This matches with how religious traditions emphasize the importance of the intention behind selfless acts, and that giving or serving out of a genuine desire to help others is considered more virtuous than doing so for personal gain or recognition.

What's more, studies have also shown that people derive satisfaction from ensuring fair outcomes, even if it means a personal cost. This suggests that our brains are wired to prioritize not only our own well-being but also the well-being of others.

And at the end of life that is what patients talk about: their relationships with others. I have seen it carry my patients through their good times and their most challenging times. The often-cited Harvard Study of Adult Development, which followed Harvard men from the time they were sophomores during the Great Depression in 1938 into their eighties and nineties, found that overwhelmingly people's close relationships—the ones in which love was most likely to play a role—were the greatest predictors of meaning, happiness, and satisfaction late in life. In a separate study, researchers found that marital satisfaction helps protect people's mental health well into old age. People who had happy marriages in their eighties reported that their moods didn't suffer even on the days when they had more physical pain. Those who had unhappy marriages felt both more emotional and physical pain.

I have seen many life partners and spouses who come to medical visits together. When they arrive in my office, I see how their support of each other helps to fortify and lift each other up. One particular couple, Lisa and Bob, both of whom are my patients, remind me of this every time I see them.

Lisa has had a relatively straightforward medical journey; we are managing some of her chronic cardiovascular risk factors, but thankfully she has not suffered any cardiac events such as a heart attack or stroke. She is working hard to lower her weight, cholesterol, and blood pressure, but her biggest struggle has been staying strong for her husband, Bob. Unlike Lisa, Bob has suffered quite a few serious medical travails, including recurrent bouts of colon cancer that have had him in and out of the hospital for years without much peace. The cancer continues to come back despite his medical team's best efforts to cure him. In addition to this, he has heart disease and several other health conditions.

I have watched Bob respond resiliently, despite all of these burdens, with Lisa's support. It helps that he has a great sense of humor, and the two laugh together a lot. This past year after Bob suffered a fall, he was hospitalized with neurological issues. When I saw him after this accident, sadly he was a shadow of his prior self—he seemed weaker, smaller, and cognitively changed. His neurology team remained optimistic that despite these alarming changes, recovery back to his baseline was possible.

At their first visit together in my office after Bob left the hospital from the fall, Lisa sat in the corner of the exam room fighting back tears. At prior visits she would be listening, joking with Bob, and staying positive for him. This time she was crying, but doing her best to hide it. The man she loved, the one who'd made us all laugh, was still there inside, but the events of the last few months had taken a toll on them both. As I handed her the tissue box, we spoke of their love and of allowing for time to help them both find their way back to their baseline.

Several months later I saw Lisa and Bob at another visit and was thrilled to see that Bob was again back to cracking jokes and behaving more like his old self. He was planning for yet another procedure for his colon cancer but, as always, was facing his every challenge with grace and humor. I looked at Lisa and said, "He's back." She smiled. But I saw her eyes fill with tears, too, what I knew were both tears of joy at his recovery, and tears of grief because she was still suffering each day watching the man she loved fight so hard to survive for both of them.

Their love is just one story of so many I have watched as a physician. I have seen how love can be a medicine that is just as powerful if not more so than the kind that we give as pills or infusions. I believe the power of love can also literally pull us back from the brink of death.

I recently watched the documentary *Super/Man: The Christopher Reeve Story*, about the aftermath of the accident that left the world-famous actor paralyzed from the neck down in 1995. When he was lying motionless in a hospital bed, realizing that life as he knew it was over, he started to doubt whether he wanted to continue. If it weren't for the love of his wife, Dana, he is sure he would have made a different choice. In the film he recalls:

> Dana came into the room; she knelt down next to me and we made eye contact. And then I mouthed my first lucid words to her: "Maybe we should let me go."
>
> Dana started crying and she said, "I'm only going to say this once. I'll support whatever you want to do because this is your life and your decision. But I want you to know I'll be with you for the long haul, no matter what."
>
> And then she added the words that saved my life: "You're still you and I love you."

The Healing Power of Resilience

I think if she had looked away or paused or hesitated even slightly or if I had felt there was a sense of her being noble, I don't know if I could have pulled through.

Christopher subsequently elaborated, "When Dana whispered those lifesaving words to me, 'You're still you and I love you,' it meant more to me than just a personal declaration of faith and commitment. In a sense it was an affirmation that marriage and family stood at the center of everything, and if both were intact, so was your universe."

This story is remarkable to me for a few reasons, but one is to see how the love between him and his wife gave him the strength to respond resiliently at his lowest point. At that moment, he felt that love from her was all there was, all that truly mattered, at the center of his universe. Equally astounding to me is that Dana loved him enough to allow that he might choose to die—and that she was ready to take on suffering to relieve him of his.

After his accident, Christopher and Dana became prominent advocates for spinal-cord-injury research and disability rights. Together they founded the Christopher & Dana Reeve Foundation, "dedicated to curing spinal cord injury by advancing innovative research and improving the quality of life for individuals and families impacted by paralysis." The two worked together tirelessly to improve the quality of life for people with a range of disabilities. Ten months after Christopher died from sepsis in October of 2004 at the age of fifty-two, Dana was diagnosed with a lung cancer that ultimately took her life only a year and a half later. She was only forty-four years old.

When we talk about love, we should also talk about grief. Grief, like love, is difficult to define, but one definition that resonates with me is offered by Dr. Katherine Shear, professor of psychiatry at Columbia

University School of Social Work. She calls grief "the form that love takes when someone we love dies."

We have all heard people say "I can't live without" someone, but apparently for some this is actually true. In a medical phenomenon called the widowhood effect, a surviving spouse is more likely to die relatively recently to their partner's passing than is someone who has not suffered the loss of a spouse. A study conducted by the Harvard School of Public Health found the increased chance of dying after a spouse dies is greatest in the first three months after the loss, when the surviving spouse has a 66 percent increased chance of dying. Even more astounding, a 2014 study in *JAMA Internal Medicine* showed that within thirty days of a partner's death, people who were sixty and older had more than twice the risk of a stroke or heart attack compared to those who hadn't suffered the death of a spouse. This added to a study several years before by the American Heart Association that showed the danger of a heart attack was highest in the first twenty-four hours after the death of a loved one, and people with existing cardiovascular problems seemed to be at particular risk.

The reasons for these phenomena are complex. Often, the stress response kicks in after a deep loss. Dr. Lisa M. Shulman, professor of neurology at the University of Maryland School of Medicine, said much of the physical effect of grief stems from this stress. As Dr. Shulman explains, "Your heart starts racing, your blood pressure increases, your respiratory rate increases, you become sweaty, as the body prepares to protect itself." This physiological response can be triggered by reminders of the loss—for example, upon entering the bedroom of the person who died, or even when someone mentions the person's name. Often, people don't understand why they're having such a strong reaction. "Instead, you just feel this incredible physiologic response and a rising sense of anxiety, or even panic. And you're flummoxed by it," says Shulman. If this grief-induced stress becomes chronic, like any other stress the cascading effect it creates can be detrimental to health in a whole host of ways.

Losing a spouse can take a significant toll on physical health in other ways, too. Grief can weaken our immune system, making us more susceptible to illness. Exhaustion caused by insomnia or restlessness can exacerbate existing or underlying health conditions. In addition, bereavement often disrupts daily routines and habits. A surviving spouse may experience disrupted patterns in sleep, appetite, and exercise, all of which can negatively impact their health. They may also neglect their own health needs, doing such things as skipping doctors' appointments, forgetting to take medications, or neglecting preventive care. The death of a spouse can also lead to social isolation and loneliness, especially if the partner was a primary source of companionship and support. When you combine all of these factors, grief can be a heavy load to bear indeed.

Dr. Shulman's interest in the neurobiology of grief is personal. Following the death of her husband, fellow neurobiologist Dr. Bill Weiner, from cancer, she experienced the disorientation and confusion that often accompany profound loss. Despite her professional experience with grieving patients, she said she felt unprepared for the reality of her grief.

The first two years were especially challenging, when she felt as if she were living every day in a fog—a common dissociative response to intense emotional pain. Shulman withdrew from the world and slid down the slippery slope of isolating, which further compounded the pain of grieving. She needed to call upon and build up several components of her Resilience Response to get through the pain and on the road to healing. And she did. After accepting the hard fact of her loss, she turned to mindfulness and relaxation practices, journaling, cognitive behavior therapy, and, finally, seeking out connection with others through writing her book, *Before and After Loss: A Neurologist's Perspective on Loss, Grief, and Our Brain.* She now speaks regularly on the topics of grief and neuroplasticity. The ability to share her experiences, recognize commonality with others, and have open conversations about grief have helped her to move forward in her life.

Love and the Heart

We know that grief affects the brain and the body. But humans respond to grief in a variety of ways. In some cases the unexpected death of a loved one or other extreme emotional stress (such as that caused by an acute illness, a serious accident, or a natural disaster) can trigger a temporary weakening of the heart muscle, mimicking a heart attack. This is known as broken heart syndrome or, more scientifically, stress cardiomyopathy or takotsubo cardiomyopathy. Japanese investigators noted that during this type of attack the enlarged left ventricle of the heart looks similar to a *takotsubo* pot, a Japanese device used to catch octopus, thus the unusual terminology.

This peculiar type of heart attack is not caused by the common culprits such as narrowed arteries or other blockages of blood vessels, or from any type of rupture of plaque or muscle. Instead it is caused by an incredible surge of adrenaline that can accompany extreme emotional distress. As Dr. Howard Lewine, internist at Brigham and Women's Hospital in Boston, explains, this surge can "essentially 'stun' the heart, triggering changes in heart muscle cells or coronary blood vessels (or both) that prevent the left ventricle from contracting effectively." More than 90 percent of total reported cases of stress cardiomyopathy are in women, and 80 percent of those cases appear in females over the age of fifty. While usually not fatal, this condition highlights the incredibly powerful connection between grief and health.

Despite how bad stress and its accompanying hormonal activity can be for all of our bodily systems, not all hormonal surges do damage to the heart. We know the hormone, oxytocin, actually promotes heart health.

Oxytocin, as we've discussed, is associated with pleasure and stress reduction; it is also associated with childbirth (it stimulates uterine contractions) and breastfeeding (it promotes milk production and release). It also plays a role in sexual arousal for both men and women as well as delivering what athletes call a runner's high. Acts of kindness, such as volunteering, helping others, or simply expressing compassion, also stimulate the release of oxytocin. This release has been shown to reduce stress, lower blood pressure, and promote feelings of relaxation and well-being. Oxytocin incites feelings of trust, safety, and connection, and it's rather unique among hormones in that it can also stimulate a sense of exhilarating calm. (Altruistic behavior can also activate the brain to release dopamine, another neurotransmitter, which is associated with pleasure, motivation, and feelings of satisfaction.)

One of the primary ways to stimulate oxytocin release is through touch. Perhaps this is why it's been dubbed the love hormone, as it draws us together and is released when we hug, cuddle, and enjoy sex. We all know that touch is a powerful means of connecting with others or conveying meaning. But the degree of emotional nuance that can be conveyed in this way is astounding. Touch is a method of communication that can be as useful as speech. In a 2009 study, researchers found that touch can successfully communicate a whole host of emotions including anger, fear, happiness, sadness, disgust, love, gratitude, and sympathy.

Physical touch isn't the only way to calm or soothe us, but it is particularly potent and fast acting. A 2021 study of 159 participants showed that a soothing touch or hug reduces cortisol responses to psychosocial stress. Holding hands with a loved one, experiencing "supportive touch" during a painful procedure has been proven to lessen the perception of pain. Additional studies have also shown that physical touch can lower levels of cortisol, reducing anxiety, improving mood, and lead to a stronger immune system. That's because physical touch causes our brain to release the chemical signals that can correct the physiological dysregulation caused by the stress of loneliness and return us to equilibrium.

Though the skin is perhaps the most obvious organ involved in the release of oxytocin in the body, new research shows there are oxytocin receptors in the vessels and chambers of the human heart. There, oxytocin is known to act as a hypotensive agent, meaning it lowers and helps regulate blood pressure. It also increases the production of chemicals that dilate and open the blood vessels, helping blood move freely through the body.

Recent research at Michigan State University shows that oxytocin, when administered after cardiac injury (such as a heart attack), promotes the regeneration of epicardial cells. (It is important to note that this does not mean that the injured heart muscle itself can be repaired or regenerated . . . yet.) These cells make up the epicardium, which is the outermost layer of cells covering the heart muscle, and this regeneration likely mimics the role oxytocin played in the original development of the heart. Dr. Aitor Aguirre, assistant professor of biomedical engineering at Michigan State, is one of the lead researchers on this project. He applies an engineering approach to understanding how the human heart is formed and how it responds to injury. Even though we humans don't have the capacity to regenerate our heart, other animals do—and we can learn from them to see how we might be able to scientifically develop this ability. We know already that the heart, when injured, does produce some stem cells, but not enough to have any effect on heart-cell regeneration. Aguirre and his team are conducting experiments to see if there is a way to boost this stem cell production to jump-start cardiac cellular repair, and this is where oxytocin comes into play. Their work is part of the newer science of regenerative medicine, which is built around the belief that since the body once produced the basic cells (what we call stem stems) needed to create an organ wholesale, it likely has the capacity to produce enough of those cells to repair that organ. Aguirre's work with oxytocin as an agent for stimulating this kind of cell growth shows promise; perhaps medical intervention might be used to help the human body produce regenerative cells that could prevent the onset of, or even reverse, cardiovascular disease.

The Importance of Self-Love

There are other ways of getting the good hormones surging, too—things you can do all by yourself. I know that listening to me dispense advice on learning to love yourself may cause you to groan aloud. Or it may simply sound impossible if you don't feel connection, much less love, to and from the people around you. But the first step to self-love is self-compassion, which means being kind to yourself, even if you think you don't deserve it. And according to research, self-compassion itself pays dividends to health.

Self-compassion acts as a buffer against stress, promotes healthier behaviors such as regular exercise and better diet, and enhances emotional regulation, allowing us to cope with challenges more effectively (and, obviously, resiliently!). This has been proven in study after study, such as one published in the *Journal of Health Psychology*, which found that self-compassion was positively associated with various health-promoting behaviors, such as regular exercise, healthy eating, and stress management. Or another published in 2020 that showed that self-compassion was linked to lower levels of pain catastrophizing (exaggerating pain and feeling helpless) and improved emotional well-being in individuals with chronic pain.

Of particular interest to me is a study published in *Health Psychology*, in which Rebecca C. Thurston, Director of the Women's Biobehavioral Health Program at the University of Pittsburgh, and her colleagues recruited 159 women without cardiovascular disease (CVD) to see how self-compassion might be related to their medical outcomes. Thurston and her coauthors employed the Self-Compassion Scale—a test developed to assesses the subject's response to twelve different statements on a scale of 1 (almost never) to 5 (almost always). These statements range from "I try to be loving towards myself when I'm feeling emotional pain" to "When I'm feeling down, I tend to feel like most other people are probably happier than I am." Dr. Thurston found that women with greater self-compassion had a lower rate of subclinical cardiovascular disease—which is where there are signs of CVD without any symptoms. It can be an early stage of CVD that leads to stroke and other poor health outcomes. These participants with more self-compassion specifically had lower carotid intima-media thickness (IMT), which is associated with cardiovascular risk factors and is predictive of cardiovascular events.

I would call practicing self-care a first-level way you can start to demonstrate self-compassion, which can lead to a deeper sense of self-love. The World Health Organization defines self-care as "the ability of individuals, families and communities to promote their own health, prevent disease, maintain health, and to cope with illness with or without the support of a health or care worker." In other words, if you're struggling, seek out help. If you need to rest, take time for yourself. If you suspect something just isn't right, visit your doctor. A Healthy Cities initiative of WHO also identified twelve key determinants for people to be able to practice self-care, including access to services, healthy food, open spaces, safe environments, healthy air, physical activity, and social cohesion.

The research supports the decision to take care of yourself, too. In a 2017 study published in the *Journal of the American Heart Association*, Dr. Barbara Riegel and her coauthors found that practicing self-care is crucial to support the American Heart Association's mission of bringing down the rate of CVD in the United States—and that it is imperative it be built into our culture as a society. For instance, self-measuring and monitoring your blood pressure at home is correlated with a decrease in both systolic and diastolic blood pressure, more so than when blood pressure is only measured in regular medical care. Additionally, looking at cardiac rehabilitation programs, people receiving standard care were more likely to die from heart-related issues and more likely to be readmitted to the hospital or have another heart attack if they only adhered to a medical rehab program. On the flip side, lifestyle-change programs, which included self-care components such as diet and exercise, led to better results. Programs that helped people set goals, track their progress, plan ahead, and get feedback—to work on themselves holistically, with the help of others—worked best.

So where to begin? If you are feeling isolated and alone, unloved and unlovable, how can you begin to practice self-care that can lead to compassion and self-love?

Self-care is highly personal. What works for one person may not work for another. It's about identifying activities that replenish your physical, emotional, and mental resources. Here are some things that I'd suggest as places to begin.

Seek Out Love

For physical self-care, recall some of the things we talked about in taking care of your physical health—one of the cornerstones without which we can't build a sound self-love. To begin:

- Get enough sleep (seven to nine hours for most adults)
- Eat a balanced and nutritious diet as best you can
- Engage in regular physical activity (exercise, yoga, walking)
- Stay hydrated
- Take breaks during work or other activities when needed and possible

Studies show time and again that mindfulness practices can lead to significant reductions in cortisol levels. This is one way that emotional self-care can directly impact our well-being. For emotional self-care, some great ways to start are:

- Practice mindfulness or meditation. Begin by taking just five minutes a day, first thing in the morning. Try to empty your mind for quiet contemplation. A good way to do this is to focus on the sound of your breath, entering and leaving your body
- Journal or express your creativity, for instance through the arts or music
- Spend time in nature
- Engage in hobbies and activities you enjoy (reading, sports, gardening, sewing, whatever interests you or brings you joy)
- Practice setting boundaries and practicing saying no to things that drain you

- Seek therapy or counseling when needed, or as part of a process of greater self-discovery

Self-care can also be social. Seek connection, and build from there to deeper relationships. With that in mind, try to:

- Make an effort to regularly spend time with loved ones (friends, family, pets)
- Step out and connect with your community by volunteering or participating in local activities or get-togethers
- Work on building and maintaining healthy relationships, even if these begin with a casual "Hello" to the barista at your favorite coffee shop, or the coworker you always end up with in the elevator
- Practice effective communication skills—when things are easy, and when they get tougher

Self-care can also be spiritual, even if you do not adhere to any specific religion. You can:

- Connect with your values and beliefs through reflection and practice
- Spend time in reflection or prayer
- Engage in activities that bring you a sense of purpose and meaning

Self-care is a way to check in on ourselves. It gives us an opportunity to replenish our physical, emotional, and mental resources, which will better equip us to handle stress and challenges. Think of acts of self-care as charging your battery. Every time you engage in self-care, you are shoring up your energy to respond resiliently, so you'll be better prepared when the tough times come. And they will come, for all of us.

Love as an Ingredient to a Resilient Response

I was lucky enough to have a loving childhood, buffered and protected and supported by my parents and brother, and to have understood the security that comes with feeling loved. Seeking and cultivating love has always been part of my path in life, as I carried with me my favorite childhood movie line, "True love is the greatest thing in all the world," from *The Princess Bride*. Despite this, I made many wrong choices and turns throughout my early twenties and thirties. Not until the age of thirty-four when I met my husband, David, did I learn and feel and understand real love. When we first started dating, he told me I was his lobster, referring to an episode of the TV show *Friends* when one of the characters says, "It's a known fact that lobsters fall in love and mate for life. You can actually see old lobster couples, walking around their tank, you know, holding claws."

Before we got married, a close friend advised me that the words "love, trust, and empower" each other should define our union, and I do believe those words are a beautiful map of what loving relationships are built on. She went on to say she believed we would do more together on this planet than we could ever do apart. And we have.

David's love and our love have allowed me to grow in a million ways. It also brought me our amazing two daughters. Through them, my understanding of the limitless capacity for love has grown even more. The love I share with my children is hard to capture in words, but it feels like an endless infinity loop that ties us together.

The Healing Power of Resilience

I am lucky to have witnessed this many times through the experiences of my patients, such as Bob and Lisa, and their own children as well. Many times it is the love of their children that has pushed my patients to take control of their health. I hear them say they only began to prioritize their health so they could be present for a child's graduation or wedding, or simply to be there for their children as they progress through the travails of life.

The love that courses through the parent-child bond is powerful, too. Through our conversations in the exam rooms I have heard mothers and fathers speak of the pain and suffering they endure watching their children struggle through mental health issues, addiction, terminal illness. I see the toll it takes on the parents—but also know the load feels so heavy precisely because of the strength of love that binds them. On the other side, I have seen children who bring their parents to each visit with me, diligently taking notes, scheduling testing, and making sure their parents are managed medically. And in those last moments, I have watched as children huddle at the ICU bedside of their parents saying their last goodbyes; telling their parents it's okay to let go and be at peace. The love, in every case, is a source of support from which patients and their loved ones can respond resiliently.

Love is visible in these big moments of support, but I often think of the importance in our lives of the little moments of love—the hugs in the hallway, the texts that say "I'm thinking of you," the bedtime whispers of "I love you" before we close our eyes at night, the small gestures that mean so much. I think of this often with my youngest daughter. When she was little, my sister-in-law, who is a child psychologist, gave us a book called *The Invisible String*, about the powerful bonds that connect us to others. My daughter and I often speak about the string that connects us always and forever, even when we are apart. We tell

Seek Out Love

each other to "remember our string," and as we say goodbye for the day, we roll our hands to reel in the string and say, "Do you feel me tugging on it?" One day when I came to work, I found a sticky note in my bag from my daughter that said, "I love you, and I'm pulling on your string." These tiny notes are powerful daily reminders of our relationship. I encourage my patients to think about the little ways to foster love in their own lives.

The bottom line: Allow yourself to love and be loved. Make finding it, fostering it, growing it, a priority, just as you would eating a healthy diet or exercising or getting enough sleep. Love is not only the best medicine; it is truly the elixir of life.

Even as I write this, I feel my nervous system relax and my heart open to the realization that the more we love and care for one another, the more support and care we give and get from one another, the more resilient we can be. If resilience propels us to move forward in life in the face of both everyday and extraordinary challenges, it has no more powerful a fuel than love.

CHAPTER 9

Finding Hope and Having Faith

Sometimes, a health event can be so scary that a patient can't believe another day will come. Sometimes, a diagnosis can be so dire that a patient can't imagine what the next day will look like. When we learn we don't have much future left, or if what lies ahead looks completely unlike the life we have known so far . . . what happens next?

That's when we need hope the most. Hope is the foundation that allows us to build a Resilience Response in the moment, whatever happens next.

My feelings on hope and how important it is for medical care are well illustrated through a lesson I learned in my third year of medical school, when I attended a lecture by one of the hematologist/oncologist attendings, Dr. Alexandra Levine. She relayed a story from when she was in training, shadowing a senior physician on rounds. When they came to a patient recovering from cancer surgery, the senior doctor said aloud that this person's chance of long-term survival was little to none. Within days of that conversation the patient died. Dr. Levine told us that while the patient did have a late-stage cancer and faced a difficult course of treatment, nothing indicated they could not have survived at least one to five years or more. The doctor took hope away from the patient through the prognosis, and the patient lost the will to live. Dr. Levine conveyed loud and clear the message she wanted to share with us: *Never take hope away from a patient.*

I have always remembered her words and think of them every time I speak to one of my patients about a new diagnosis. Hope is infused in every conversation I have around the future of his or her care. A line from one of my favorite movies, *The Shawshank Redemption*, goes "Hope is a good thing, maybe the best of things, and no good thing ever dies." I hold fast to this idea when giving hard news.

Countless times I have witnessed patients beat the odds and live beyond expectations—even if it was a stretch to think they would survive just one more day. For many it is that one more day, and that one more day has so much value for them and the people who love them. Allowing for hope is a key part of how we can help people and patients build resilience. Instead of limiting our expectations of what happens next to fit within the smallest, safest perimeter, we should allow people the room to grow, to live into whatever might be possible.

Hope is difficult to define; we just know it when we feel it. One definition of hope that I like defines it as an "optimistic state of mind based on the expectation of positive outcomes in one's life or the world." This means to me that hope is something we can choose to cultivate. Hope is a positive motivational state based on a sense of agency (the belief that you can initiate and direct actions) and action (the belief that you can find ways to achieve your goals). It's not simply wishful thinking; it's a belief in the possibility of a better future, coupled with the conviction that you can play a role in making that future a reality. If we believe that resilience is, rather than the ability to bounce back, the ability to bounce forward and to find peace with a new normal, hope is believing that we can make that new normal a good place to be.

On the other hand, the absence of hope is something that can more easily be quantified and analyzed, often via the Beck Hopelessness Scale. This self-reporting tool was developed in the 1980s by leading psychiatrist Dr. Aaron Beck, widely regarded as the pioneer of cognitive behavioral therapy. It asks a person to answer true or false to questions such as "I might as well give up because I can't make things better for myself," "I don't expect to get what I really want," "In the future, I expect to succeed in what concerns me most," and "My past experiences have prepared me well for the future." A score is assessed and the respondent is placed on a scale that determines the level and immediacy of intervention required. The scale is often used with people at risk for depression and suicide, but it can be useful in other settings as well.

We're trying to get better at measuring hope, such as through the use of the Adult Hope Scale (AHS), which was developed slightly more recently, in 1991, by C. R. Snyder, distinguished professor of clinical psychology at the University of Kansas. Snyder's theory of hope is that it is a stable trait related to goal pursuit, built upon two components: pathways and agency. Pathways refer to a person's ability to see a way forward toward a goal and whether they can come up with a plan to achieve it. Agency means that a person believes that they have the capacity to do so—they either believe they already intrinsically possess what it takes to reach their goal, or that they can learn or acquire the needed skills. Building on this concept of hope, Snyder created a self-report measure of hope, the AHS. It has been used in studies ranging from academic outcomes, to lung-cancer symptoms, to visual impairment, to marital status, to suicidal ideation. Research into hope's relationship with health-related outcomes is of special interest to me, as it gives us insight into hope-related interventions that can be used by medical practitioners to help our patients improve their physical and mental health.

As I learned more about Snyder's work, I read a remarkable remembrance of him as a doctor and a person in the forward to *The Oxford Handbook of Positive Psychology.* The book was edited by Snyder and one of his protégés, psychologist and hope expert and research director of the Clifton Strengths Institute Shane Lopez. In the forward, Lopez recalled, "One uncommonly good man tirelessly worked to help many others become the uncommonly good people he foresaw that they could be. . . . Rick Snyder's scholarship shows us how to connect to positive future opportunities through hope." Lopez died some years later. In turn, when he himself was memorialized, a colleague recalled, "Shane was fond of speaking about the importance of spreading ripples of hope. The many scientists, practitioners, and students he inspired to have the passion and skills to study and spread hope are just one of the many ways in which Shane leaves a legacy of spreading ripples of hope to bolster the hope and well-being of those around him." Clearly, that ripple extended from mentor to mentee, and then again outward from that individual to the next generation of researchers, and it will continue to echo still further.

Snyder's foundational work helped to inspire Shane; it also furthered our understanding of the correlation between hope, or its absence, and medical outcomes. A study of nearly thirteen thousand American adults with the mean age of sixty-six published in *Global Epidemiology* in 2020 looks at the relationship between hope and physical, behavioral, and psychosocial outcomes. A few key findings: Over the four-year follow-up period, the third of participants reporting the highest level of hope had a 16 percent lower risk of all-cause mortality, 12 percent reduced probability of cancer, and 11 percent reduced probability of chronic pain. The study is significant because it not only verifies the psychological benefits of hope, but also its physiological and behavioral benefits as well. Subjects who felt hopeful reported such things as being more physically active, sleeping better, and having a better overall general sense of well-being.

Another study published in 2020 in the *Journal of Advanced Nursing* looked at thirty-three English and Dutch studies conducted over the previous decade to examine the role hope plays in the lives of cancer patients. Patients who felt hopeful reported a higher overall quality of life, in spite of the type or stage of cancer they had. I take this to mean that hope is an inside job, and that we can find it within ourselves—even when our external circumstances may seem grim. I am not, however, recommending that we encourage false or blind hope: Hope is decidedly *not* wishful thinking. Instead, I prefer to think of it as believing, of all the possible outcomes, the best one could happen.

Even in the direst of medical circumstances, hope can help. City of Hope, a renowned comprehensive cancer center located in the desert suburbs of Los Angeles, California, was founded as a free, nondenominational tuberculosis sanatorium in 1913. Not only does it have a long history of treating people with compassionate care, but it is also well-known for its cutting-edge medical research, which has resulted in breakthroughs including the development of synthetic human insulin and key cancer-fighting drugs such as Herceptin and Rituxan, both monoclonal antibody therapies released to the public in the late 1990s. The institution's credo is "There is no profit in curing the body if, in the process, we destroy the soul." Hope is at the center of patient care here.

City of Hope is committed to translating laboratory discoveries into clinical breakthroughs. This includes pioneering work in such areas as immunotherapy, gene therapy, and stem-cell transplantation, particularly for cancers and other complex diseases. But City of Hope isn't just about the latest science and treatments. It's a multidisciplinary environment where specialists from various fields collaborate to address the holistic needs of each patient, one by one. An integrated-care model ensures that each patient receives comprehensive care, meaning not only medical treatment but also such things as nutritional counseling, pain management, and psychosocial support. Because we know that physical health is linked to emotional well-being, City of Hope also provides resources and programs aimed at reducing stress, promoting mental health, and enhancing the coping mechanisms of its patients, since managing the side effects of treatment is crucial for maintaining patients' strength and quality of life. The center's focus on compassionate care also acknowledges the emotional and spiritual toll of cancer, and through education and support programs, City of Hope helps people mount a Resilience Response in the face of serious illness.

Alexandra Levine, the doctor I mentioned studying with earlier, is a distinguished figure at City of Hope. After working with Dr. Jonas Salk on AIDS vaccine development and serving on the Presidential Advisory Council on HIV/AIDS, Dr. Levine served as chief medical officer at City of Hope for nearly a decade, overseeing all aspects of patient care, quality of service, and clinical research. She is now a professor in the department of hematology and hematopoietic cell transplantation where she works at the forefront of our understanding and treatment of lymphoma, Hodgkin's disease, and AIDS-related malignancies.

City of Hope's CEO, Dr. Michael Friedman, who hired Levine in 2006, saw that she fosters hope in the way she cares for patients—by embodying it in her treatment of them. "There have been countless moments by a touch, by an expression, by just the inclination of her

Finding Hope and Having Faith

body, she indicated a deep devotion to the care of that individual and established a kind of linkage with the patient and the family that was sort of magical to watch," Friedman said. I was lucky enough to witness this firsthand in my medical studies.

I've noticed that teachers who have become my mentors all put hope at the center of their practices. I had the chance recently to interview another of my mentors, Dr. Astrid Heger. Dr. Heger emphasizes the importance of hope in the work she does with severely abused children and young adults. She told me one story I will never forget. She recalled that in 1999, a tough case was referred to her at her practice in Los Angeles—she was asked by the FBI to help in the treatment of a girl named Jennifer who had been made a sex slave in Hong Kong and trafficked to the United States. When Dr. Heger met her, the young woman had a tough demeanor and was not open to treatment. Dr. Heger did her best to break through to her, but could not. And after just a few weeks Jennifer was sent back to Hong Kong to her parents because she was a minor.

Later, Dr. Heger was subpoenaed to testify in the case against the man who coerced Jennifer into sex slavery. She had to fly to Hong Kong to testify in Jennifer's case. In the courtroom, the narrative advanced was that this girl was a seductress, that she'd asked for it, and on and on. Even her parents were visibly angered with her; they wouldn't go near her. And Jennifer stood there sobbing on the stand, at fourteen years old.

Eventually the man who coerced her into sex slavery was sentenced to one year in prison. One year. As Dr. Heger left the courtroom, in a rush to catch her plane back to the United States, she saw Jennifer standing in the foyer outside the courtroom, alone. Still sobbing. Dr. Heger told me. "So I walk over, put my arms around her, and say, 'What they said about you in there is not true. You can be anything you want. When you're older, you can come back to LA. I'm right there. You come

The Healing Power of Resilience

find me. I'll be there for you.'" I was moved by Dr. Heger's story. She explained, "[I] just gave her five minutes of my time, went and caught my airplane, came back to LA, figured I'd never see her again."

But the hope that Dr. Heger had shared and planted in that fourteen-year-old girl took root. Ten years later, Dr. Heger received a letter at her office. She read, "You probably don't remember me, but I'm now a grad student at UCLA. And when you stopped, you changed my life." It was from Jennifer, who, thanks to that interaction, had responded resiliently and moved forward in her life in a way no one could ever have anticipated. "It was five minutes of my time. And if I had missed my plane, it would've been well worth those five minutes." Those five minutes gave Jennifer the hope she needed to choose a completely different future for herself.

I try to think about how I can make space for those five minutes with my patients. I want each of them to feel hopeful when they leave my office. I see this especially in a few—they are the ones that I joke have nine lives. These are individuals who have been through more medical diagnosis and issues than you would think one person could tolerate, but yet they keep going and keep on living. Jeff was one such patient of mine. I treated him for heart disease in the past, along with several other conditions—and then a few years ago, he was diagnosed with pancreatic cancer. He needed a complex and invasive surgery and was in the hospital recovering for months. He lost a significant amount of weight and had to rebuild from being frail and fragile back into the athlete he was before the cancer. Jeff is also a triathlete, and a business owner, and despite all of his health challenges, I've seen him recover time after time and get back to training and to work. Not once have I seen him knocked down by any of the challenges he has faced. He always has a hopeful outlook that I find so inspiring, and I am convinced that is part of how he has responded so resiliently to so many challenges.

Faith

I love how clinical psychologist Anthony Scioli defines hope as "an emotion with spiritual dimensions," because it so beautifully gets at the undefinable, mystical power of hope.

This connects hope to a closely related but distinct sentiment, or some might call it a practice: faith. Faith, from a psychological and scientific perspective, is a complex phenomenon that extends beyond traditional religious contexts. It encompasses a deep-seated belief in something unseen, a conviction that transcends empirical evidence. It involves a trust in a higher power, a set of principles, or even in your own capabilities, which can then act as a powerful coping mechanism and source of strength during times of stress and uncertainty. We've found that faith can activate neural pathways associated with reward and positive emotions, contributing to feelings of well-being. Belief in a treatment's efficacy can lead to real, measurable physiological changes, demonstrating the mind's capacity to influence the body, as we discussed in regard to the placebo effect.

When someone's faith takes the form of a religious practice, it often becomes intertwined with communal support, rituals, and moral codes. These elements help to reduce social isolation and provide a structured framework for navigating life's challenges. Many studies, including one meta-analysis that covered a period of over fifty years, published in the journal *Depression Research and Treatment,* have shown that regular attendance at religious services is associated with lower rates of depression and anxiety. In this study, increased religious attendance predicted a 49 percent lower likelihood of mood disorder, and 53 percent lower likelihood of any psychiatric disorder. Attendance also reduced the effect that parental depression had on children: For high-risk children, those who had depressed parents and also had high exposure to negative life events, religious attendance reduced the likelihood of major depression by 76 percent. Research has also demonstrated that religious coping strategies, such as prayer and meditation, can also help individuals manage chronic pain and improve their overall quality of life. A study published in the *American Journal of Epidemiology* found that individuals who attended religious services more than once a week had a 33 percent lower risk of mortality than those who didn't.

Most doctors stay away from discussions about spirituality or religion with patients. But thankfully, it appears there is a growing awareness of the positives of linking healthcare and spirituality: The number of medical schools offering courses on related subjects increased from 13 percent in 1994 to around 90 percent in 2010. Though I never impose any of my personal beliefs or opinions on the topic when I care for patients, I do participate in a dialogue with those in my care about religion and spirituality if they so choose. I like to use the HOPE acronym, developed by doctors at Brown University School of Medicine: The *H* prompts doctors to ask about sources of hope and strength, the *O* addresses connection to organized religion, the *P* touches on personal spiritual practices, and the *E* refers to the effects of spirituality on medical care.

I've seen firsthand how a patient's beliefs can play a role in treatment and its effectiveness. It may sound counterintuitive, but sometimes it takes getting sick to realize just how good we have it. Illness can shift our awareness toward recognition and appreciation of all that we have, and the realization that we may—and will—lose it all one day. Our days are limited, though we sometimes have a hard time remembering this and behaving as such.

Finding Hope and Having Faith

One case of mine where I saw this play out firsthand was in a sixty-three-year-old woman whom I saw for a cardiac evaluation after she was diagnosed with breast cancer. At first she didn't want aggressive intervention, but then chose to have a mastectomy, chemo, and radiation. I noticed a small cross she wore and asked her about it. She pointed upward and said, "I am not alone on this journey." Her faith helped her maintain hope during treatment—and six months later, she was cancer-free.

Sometimes faith leads a person down a different path. I've had cases with people who are diagnosed with heart failure but do not want to have a defibrillator implanted or some other intervention, which they deem as interfering with God's or some other higher power's decision as to when it's "time to go."

Beyond my own experience, there's the data: It turns out that people are often eager to discuss HOPE, and their faith and spirituality, in a clinical setting. In one study combining the results conducted in the waiting room of five different family-medicine practices, 83 percent of patients were willing to discuss spiritual beliefs (63 percent depending on the situation and 20 percent always). The more critical people's medical situation, the more apt they were to desire such a conversation. A different study of 162 parents of children in pediatric intensive care found that 34 percent would like their physician to inquire about their spiritual/religious views. The number increased to 48 percent if the child was seriously ill.

Another study documented the top three reasons people reported wanting such a discussion were "so that the doctor can understand how your beliefs influence how you deal with being sick," "so that the doctor can understand you better," and "so that the doctor would understand how you make decisions." Unfortunately, despite these desires, patients are rarely asked about their religious or spiritual beliefs.

It appears that those with faith or who consider themselves to be spiritual might be better off when confronted with a difficult diagnosis or battling disease. As mentioned previously, studies have shown time and time again that those who participate in organized religion, engage in some kind of spiritual practice, or just have faith do have better health outcomes than those who don't. In a review of studies about the relationship between faith and health, Dr. Harold Koenig found that faith leads to better health outcomes. Furthermore, the data reveals that having a spiritual practice or mental framework to lean on lessens anxiety and depression among patients when compared to those who don't have religious or spiritual beliefs.

Drs. Tracy Balboni, Tyler VanderWeele, and Howard Koh are the cochairs of the Interfaculty Initiative on Health, Spirituality, and Religion at Harvard. When they dug into the research on spirituality, they found that faith wasn't just helpful in preventing negative health outcomes—it was integral. They found that neglecting to ask a patient about his or her spiritual framework was a missed opportunity. That in patient-centered care, understanding what helps the patient actually . . . helps the patient. As Koh put it, "Overlooking spirituality leaves patients feeling disconnected from the health care system and the clinicians trying to care for them. Integrating spirituality into care can help each person have a better chance of reaching complete well-being and their highest attainable standard of health."

But there can be a flip side to religious and spiritual beliefs, too, when it comes to health and well-being. Some religions doubt or denounce the efficacy or appropriateness of some aspects of Western medicine or certain treatment modalities. And this can complicate treatment planning, such as when a religious objection arises to a lifesaving blood transfusion for a child, for instance. As doctors, we might know and be able to implement a treatment to save a patient's life, and if it goes against a patient's religious beliefs, they might refuse it—with the end result being death. This is especially heart-wrenching when a parent denies a treatment for their child, as is within their protected rights. But the research shows that the benefits of a religious or spiritual orientation, including having a faith-based community to support you, outweigh the negatives.

I've seen some of my patients, those who have a rich spiritual life, approach treatment with a kind of peaceful acceptance that allows them to take the first step in the Resilience Response. With others, especially those who may struggle with a tough diagnosis or a challenging outcome, I see them lean into their spiritual beliefs as a source of both support and comfort while they find their way to acceptance. Whether one's faith is rock-solid or it emerges at the moment of crisis, it is a valuable asset in health and well-being.

One patient of mine whose faith has carried her through is Denielle Loprete. Fifteen years ago, she had no idea that her occasional bouts of fainting and exhaustion were actually sick sinus syndrome, a heart-rhythm disorder that required her to have a pacemaker implanted in her heart. The surgery went well, she recovered fully, and she resumed her work as the director of a dance studio as she parented three girls and cared for her aging father. She had regular tests, which on one fateful day in 2018 revealed an almost complete blockage of her left main coronary artery.

I read the results virtually as soon as they came in as I was away on vacation with my family. I immediately picked up the phone. Denielle recalls the details of those moments with complete clarity. Two days before, she had been out celebrating the holidays with her father and one of her daughters, and they went to a special-occasion steak house and had a bottle of wine together. Later Denielle felt a strange pain in her neck, but didn't connect it to anything heart related. She admonished herself that she needed to eat better and lose some weight in the new year.

When we spoke on the phone after I received the results, she remembers me asking her, "Where are you?" And when she reported she was at home, I said, "Stay right there. I am going to call you back in five minutes. Don't go anywhere." When I called back, Denielle recalls that I told her to ask her husband to come home from work immediately and to take her directly to Lenox Hill Hospital, to ask for Dr. Singh, the interventional cardiologist. They got Denielle in immediately to open the blockage with a stent, which undoubtedly saved her life. She is so grateful that she was given more time on earth and tells me again and again that her faith is what helped her survive, recover, and continue on in life. She attends mass frequently and prays every day. And now, she includes me in her prayers: "Before I go to sleep at night, I say, 'And God bless Dr. Narula. And her husband and her two beautiful children.'" I cannot think of any greater or more special gift.

Denielle was very open about and happy to discuss her faith. But some patients are more reluctant to share their spiritual background, even if they would actually like to or would find it helpful to talk about. A spirituality inventory, also called a spiritual assessment or spiritual history, is a helpful tool to gather information about a person's spiritual beliefs, values, and practices that I believe we should be using as regularly as we do a medical inventory that asks people about such things as a history of heart disease in their family, whether they smoke, or what kind of medications they currently take—as a key and foundational component of understanding the person and the patient in front of us in the doctor's office or hospital. When conducted in a medical setting, the inventory is designed to understand the role spirituality plays in the life of the patient in relation to their health, well-being, and coping mechanisms.

The goal of a spirituality inventory is not to diagnose or treat spiritual problems. Rather, it's to understand the individual as a person and not just a patient. Recognizing the importance of spirituality in their lives and ensuring that their spiritual needs are addressed can be of great help in understanding if a patient is prepared for the challenges that lie ahead—that is, if they might respond resiliently in a health crisis.

When preparing to conduct a spiritual inventory, it's important that the healthcare provider first establish a trusting and nonjudgmental atmosphere. Spirituality is a deeply personal matter, and the patient needs to be made comfortable and assured that the inventory is voluntary, and that the information shared will be kept confidential if requested. It's also key to acknowledge that the medical caregiver is there to listen and understand, not to proselytize or impose their own beliefs.

The inventory typically uses open-ended questions to encourage the patient to share their experiences in their own words. One most commonly used template was developed by Dr. Christina Puchalski, a palliative-care and internal-medicine specialist world leader in the movement to integrate spirituality into healthcare. She is also founder and director of the George Washington Institute for Spirituality & Health (GWish). Her approach uses the rubric FICA to pose questions related to:

F—Faith, Belief, Meaning
- *"Do you consider yourself spiritual?"* or *"Is spirituality something important to you?"*
- *"Do you have spiritual beliefs, practices, or values that help you to cope with stress, difficult times, or what you are going through right now?"* (contextualize to visit)
- *"What gives your life meaning?"*

I—Importance and Influence
- *"What importance does spirituality have in your life?"*
- *"Has your spirituality influenced how you care for yourself, particularly your health?"*
- *"Does your spirituality affect your healthcare decision-making?*

C—Community
- *"Are you part of a spiritual community?"*
- *"Do you have a community of support, and how?"* For people who don't identify with a community, consider asking, *"Is there a group of people you love or are important to you?"*
- Communities such as churches, temples, mosques, families, groups of like-minded friends, or yoga or similar groups can serve as strong support systems for some patients.

A—Address/Action in Care
- *"How would you like me, as your healthcare provider, to address spiritual issues in your healthcare?"* With newer models, including diagnosing spiritual distress, *A* also refers to the "Assessment and Plan" for patient spiritual distress, needs, and resources within a treatment or care plan.

The healthcare provider's job is to capture information, yes, but also to listen attentively and empathetically, paying attention not only to what is being said but also to the patient's body language and tone. The provider may ask clarifying questions, while remaining sensitive to topics the patient may want to avoid, and refraining from making assumptions about the patient's spirituality based on their background or appearance.

The information gathered from the spirituality inventory should then be integrated into the patient's overall care plan. The provider conducting the inventory should collaborate with other members of the healthcare team, such as social workers or psychologists, to address the patient's spiritual needs and to accommodate beliefs and practices when making decisions about their care. For example, the provider may learn about dietary restrictions related to religious observances or the need to provide a quiet space for prayer or meditation. They may seek out a referral to a chaplain, spiritual counselor, or other source of spiritual guidance if the patient expresses a desire. And with permission, the information gathered from the spirituality inventory can be added to the patient's medical record, ensuring continuity of care and improving communication between doctors and other healthcare providers.

Doing all of this first requires that healthcare providers receive appropriate training and education on how to conduct spirituality inventories in a sensitive and respectful manner. Healthcare providers must also be clear about and adhere to ethical guidelines regarding patient confidentiality and respect for autonomy when conducting this sensitive work.

The rewards of such engagement and connection can be profound not only for the patient, but for the medical professional as well. I often think about the sacred space behind the exam-room door. It is a delicate and emotional place where many of my patients share with me the most vulnerable parts of their hearts and souls. They share things they don't tell anyone else, things that make them proud, scared, tearful, happy, worried—essentially human. So often my conversations with my patients have nothing to do with blood pressure, heart disease, or cholesterol, but instead with what is happening in their lives, meaning their lives as whole people, not only patients. Many times our discussions are about hope, faith, resilience. It is not lost on me how healing is not always about fixing but so often means just listening and supporting.

My mom loves to say, you never know how one small conversation or interaction with someone can help in more ways than we can possibly know. She recently recalled for me that she had run into a woman at the bank who was the mother of a kid who was a fellow classmate of mine in high school. I had lost touch with this friend over the years, and sadly he suffered from depression and died by suicide about twenty years ago. My mom went to the funeral and spoke with my former friend's mom—but the two of them, too, grew apart in the aftermath and hadn't spoken at all in many years. At their encounter at the bank, my mom asked after her and her family. As it happened, my friend's mom opened her purse and took this paper out and said, "I have had this in my handbag, in my wallet, all of these years. This is something you gave me, and it made such a difference in my life." And it was the "Plan of the Master Weaver," a poem, more like a prayer, that my mother had given to her right after the funeral, and she had carried it with her for all those years. It begins,

My life is but a weaving
Between the Lord and me,
I may not choose the colors,
He knows what they should be.
For He can view the pattern
Upon the upper side
While I can see it only
On this, the underside.
Sometimes He weaveth sorrow,

Finding Hope and Having Faith

Which seemeth strange to me;
But I will trust His judgment,
And work on faithfully. . . .

This poem describes how to think of life as a tapestry, woven by God. You don't know which thread you are. Sometimes the threads break, and you can't predict it, and you can't explain it. The message of the poem is that we don't know what will happen. We don't know what is ahead of us. There's loss and there's sadness, but there's also beauty in every life. I think back to BJ Miller and how eloquently he speaks of the liminal space between life and death, and the glimpse he got of how profoundly beautiful that space is.

My mom had paused for just a brief moment to share this poem with another person, who had then carried that message forward, relied on it for hope over many years. I have taken to heart what my mom said about those single moments that make a difference. It's hard not to, after hearing stories from the lives of my mentors—think of Jennifer—and my patients, too. I remember so many of those "one conversations" in my life. I am grateful every day to Dr. Heger, myself, for my conversations with her, at school and beyond. I truly believe in those small moments when we cross paths with others and they listen to our worries and can see beyond them—to the best possible outcome, to a future where we feel back to a baseline. When we cannot find hope for ourselves, perhaps it is these conversations that can lend it to us for a time as we find the strength to respond to life's challenges.

Whether hope comes from within us, or without—from God, the universe, a doctor, a friend—I believe it is a crucial component of the Resilience Response.

CHAPTER 10

Pursue Your Purpose

It happens to all of us. We find ourselves at a moment when the life we know and are accustomed to is suddenly, inalterably changed. It often arises unexpectedly. It may be that we don't get into the college of our dreams or land the job we have been working toward for all of our career. Or our partner of thirty years announces that she wants a divorce. Or we are diagnosed with heart disease and are told that, if we don't alter our lifestyle as quickly as possible, we run a high risk of soon having a heart attack or stroke. These moments create a sense of great vulnerability. Our sense of who we are, our identity, is called into question.

Each of us faces a moment like this in life. But instead of its being only heartbreaking or scary, it gives us a chance to decide if perhaps that mold of who we were before no longer fits. These moments that feel like fragility can also be moments of great opportunity.

What all of these "wake-up" calls offer us is the chance for introspection, to take a closer look at our priorities, and our path, and to see if they are aligned toward what we might call our purpose. To respond resiliently—to employ acceptance, a flexible mindset, a commitment to pursuing physical health, an ability to face fears, and an optimistic or hopeful outlook—we need to find something that gives our lives meaning. We need to find our *why*. The thing that gives us reason to wake up in the morning and keep on going. That helps us bounce forward.

This is no easy task, and it's even harder if we lack some of the elements I've described in the previous chapters, especially ones that feel external to us, such as social support or love. But when a person discovers their purpose, it is beautiful to behold. Of that experience, one of my favorite writers, Kahlil Gibran, writes, "Say not, I have found the path of the soul. Say rather, I have met the soul walking upon my path."

From the time I was a small child, I wanted to be a doctor. I did not find the path of medicine. I found myself as I was walking on that path to become a doctor.

When I was a child and saw someone fall and cut their leg, I was always the first to run over to put on a Band-Aid. In the classroom I loved science, mesmerized by the intricacies of the sea and space and the world around us. I was also fascinated by the body's—and the person's—ability to move on with the help of medical intervention. I loved seeing how it all worked so magically—each and every one of our systems. I remember thinking it was a miracle that we all form the way we do with everything so perfectly synced and harmonized. There are so many things that can go wrong in our biology, and yet somehow for most of us, most of the time, we are anatomically perfectly functional. I was also fascinated by how, when we become broken, ill, or damaged, science and medicine use their tools to try to give us our lives back, whether through prosthetic limbs, stem cells, surgical techniques, or body scans; it is all so miraculous to me. And there is nothing as rewarding and meaningful as participating in this and helping someone—healing someone. All of that

Pursue Your Purpose

also factors into why I wanted to write this book. I see it as a way to help people heal on a different level.

When I was young, my father revealed to me by example the wonder and beauty of being a physician. He showed me what it meant to dedicate yourself to caring for others, to embrace the mental challenge of curing, and to involve your entire spirit in healing. He would tell me stories about his electrophysiology research—writing the first books on the electrical wiring of the heart, studying animals, designing catheters, the thrill of discovery and literally creating a new field in medicine. When I was young, he was invited all over the world to lecture and teach about his research. When he was home, I would also hear him tell stories of patients he saw both in the hospital and in his office. I saw the dedication he had to his practice: the late nights, the weekends, the holidays he devoted to caring for others. I read the countless notes and cards his patients sent, thanking him for giving them their lives back when they were on the brink of dying. Once I got older, I made rounds with him in the hospital and watched how a gentle touch on the forehead or the hand made people feel safe and protected. He was an innovator, a scientist, an incredible doctor, and a healer.

I also remember him recounting the stories of how far he traveled and how hard he worked to emigrate from India and to have the privilege of helping others in this way—through the practice of medicine. He came to America in August 1963, to join an internship program in Paterson, New Jersey. His story has so much to do with resilience and also with why I am who I am and where I am today. As he tells it:

> I couldn't come with money from India because the Indian government didn't allow you to take money out because of the shortage of foreign exchange. I was entitled to bring only fifty

dollars. And I stopped in England, London, to see my cousin there, and in the process, spending on the taxi and restaurant, I spent thirty dollars.

So I was left with twenty dollars when I ended up at JFK Airport.

My plane landed from London to there at ten in the morning. And now I have no idea where Paterson is, or how to get there. So I got off the plane, got my luggage, and I asked the people, "I need to go to Paterson, New Jersey." At the airport they tell me, "Well, you need to go to Manhattan first, and then from there you go to Paterson. You take a bus from here, it'll cost you so much . . . a couple of dollars, and that'll take you to the West Side. And then you'll have to go from the West Side to the Port Authority Terminal. . . ."

I get on the right bus. Now, I have no idea how far Paterson is from Port Authority. Was it fifteen minutes, an hour, two hours . . . three days?

So I'm sitting there, and then every time the bus stopped, I would walk up to the driver and ask, "Is this Paterson?" The guy finally got sick of me and he said to me, "You sit down, I'll tell you when you get to Paterson." I told him, "I need to go to 703 Main Street, in Paterson, St. Joseph's Hospital. He said, "The bus doesn't go there, it's about a few blocks from the hospital, so I'll drop you there, and then you go." So he dropped me and I carried my heavy bag again. . . . It's about three blocks maybe. I walk into the lobby of the hospital and there's a lady at the front desk, and I said, "I need to see Dr. Lance." And by this time it's five thirty in the evening, it's a Friday.

Pursue Your Purpose

I said, "I'm supposed to be working here." The receptionist says, "Well, let me see if I can find him." So she pages him, and then luckily the guy was still there. He greeted me and says, "Well, we won't be doing anything till Monday morning, but I'm going to find somebody who will show you around." So he got another intern to come to take me around, show me the room, and where to eat, and that was the beginning.

I didn't step out of the hospital until I got my first paycheck. I slept in the call rooms. My breakfast, lunch, and dinner, I ate them all in the hospital, hospital food. And the worst part is, I was vegetarian. So my lunch, and breakfast, were essentially the same. I would have either cheese . . . grilled-cheese sandwich or . . . I didn't used to eat eggs, then I started having eggs. So eggs, and grilled-cheese sandwich essentially . . . so I was living on that.

But I started immediately taking care of patients the right way. And each day, I would go to the library, read everything. . . . I would just voraciously read so that my informational knowledge would be great. And within a month, people realized I was smart, knowledgeable, hardworking. It gave me confidence and greater responsibility. Because I felt I had a great responsibility for patients' lives, I had to make the right decisions. So I think for my personality, that worked very well. I had the confidence after getting myself all the way there to say, "This show is mine, I need to do it right."

My salary was, I think, two hundred dollars a month. I started saving every penny. I didn't have a car. I was lonely, I had no friends. . . . I had some classmates of mine working in New York. I would take a bus, which cost me a dollar to go there and a dollar to come back, over the weekends to visit. And after about six months, I rented an apartment across the street for eighty dollars a month. I didn't have furniture. In the back of the hospital was a place where they threw away the stuff they didn't use. So I picked up a discarded hospital bed, an old mattress, an old pillow from there; they gave me pots and pans for free. I would bring a salt and pepper shaker from the hospital, and I picked up a rocking chair, a torn sofa from there, and broken chairs and tables. . . .

But people were wonderful to me. The doctors took me in. Every single doctor invited me to their home, which was unusual because I was a stranger. And then the same thing for holidays. For Thanksgiving, Christmas, on all the holidays, they would say, "We want you to come to my house." And then another would say, "I'll have him for Thanksgiving," "I'll have him for Christmas," "I'll have him for New Year's." The doctors will do that. And there was one doctor, who was really nice, he kind of adopted me. . . . Winter hadn't come when I arrived there, I had no warm clothes, so he took me shopping to buy an overcoat and things that I needed. We remained close over the years. He came to our wedding. That friendship . . . the difficulties that you go through actually make you a better person; they make you stronger, they make you more grateful for what you have and what you get from people. You gain just as much as you lose.

In fact, I felt obligated to him for what he had done. When he got sick in his older age and I could tell he was not being managed properly by his cardiologist, he needed a good cardiologist. So I had his records, reviewed them, and talked to his doctors, and he was hospitalized. I flew there to see him, to take care of him and tell them what to do with him, and then came back. I visited him twice before he died. So I felt good about it, that I was able to do something for him. Even now I maintain a friendship with his daughter.

In high school I began to follow in my father's footsteps as a healthcare practitioner when I volunteered to do research and make hospital visits in cardiac surgery. It was then that I felt the thrill of being involved in something so meaningful. Witnessing Anne's heart transplant firsthand taught me how precious and extraordinary life is. To see life pass from one person, through the hands of physicians, into another human being was nothing short of miraculous. At that moment I understood that the knowledge of how to save a life was special and sacred. I wanted to have that knowledge, too.

But despite this calling, as I mentioned earlier, I didn't pursue the straight and traditional path of studying premed as an undergrad and then going to medical school. Instead, I explored other interests. I've always had an entrepreneurial spirit, and that's why I decided to study business and start my own company. I was thoroughly devoted to it, but I also always knew that I would find way more fulfillment, meaning, and purpose in practicing medicine. Finally I couldn't ignore my yearning any longer. The more successful my company became, the more aware I was that something important was missing. I lacked the sense of fulfillment, excitement, and purpose that my early encounters with medicine had shown me. I felt lost, until I found myself on a new path—one that required a bit of backtracking, by pursuing medical school several years later than most applicants. This path has taken me to my heart's home.

The Healing Power of Resilience

But there have been forks along the way. One was exploring a dream of being a medical journalist. This passion for combining science and communication also started young—one of my favorite classes in high school was English, thanks to my fantastic teacher, Mrs. Proenza, who made me believe my words—what I had to say and how I said it—mattered. Another champion of my writing has always been my mom. She kept my journals as I progressed through school and through life, even secretly sending one of my teenage pieces off to a medical-writing competition in total secrecy—which lasted until I won.

While in medical school, I figured out pretty quickly that I didn't want to do research or have a traditional academic medical career. Yes, I wanted to help heal people, and I wanted a clinical practice. But I also decided I wanted to be a storyteller of science. I wanted to communicate the latest findings in an understandable, relatable way that made an impact, a public-health impact. I remember telling my classmates I wanted to be the next Sanjay Gupta. At that time, years ago, he was the only medical correspondent on TV. My friends in med school thought I was crazy. But that dream stayed with me throughout my training.

In my last year of cardiology fellowship in NYC, I sent my résumé to probably every magazine, TV show, and news outlet that existed. Not one place responded to my cold calls and emails except *NBC Nightly News*. They offered me an "internship," even though they had never had a doctor as an intern before. Typically the position was filled by college students. I didn't care. I was thrilled. I spent one day each week for a year trekking in to Rockefeller Center, walking through those grand doors and taking the elevator to the fourth floor, eager as I walked into the massive studio to learn everything I possibly could about the news.

When I finished my cardiology fellowship and my NBC internship in 2010, I took my very first job as an attending physician at Lenox

Pursue Your Purpose

Hill Hospital. I went to the PR office and I said, "Listen, I have this interest in medical journalism. If you need anyone to comment on any news-outlet studies, please send it my way." At first it was "Oh, there's a new study coming out about salt. Can you give some comments for the website?" Or, "It's heart-health-awareness month . . ." Little by little, I did some Web pieces. Then it was local TV. And then one day *CBS Evening News* asked if I would do a segment on heart attacks. The producer there liked me, and she introduced me to the morning producer. One thing led to another and I joined CBS News in 2014, became their senior medical correspondent in 2020, and then joined CNN—yes, where Sanjay Gupta works. The twenty-six-year-old girl in med school who dreamed about this job was suddenly on the same network as my idol. Now I work as chief medical correspondent for ABC News, which has given me the opportunity to report on and teach the public about groundbreaking research and important news in health and science—and to combine my loves of science, public health, education, and patient care. I am helping to improve not only people's health but also their health literacy—which then gives them the power to interpret and understand health information they receive about themselves, and society. My work in media has allowed me to practice medicine and also to educate, advocate, and guide. Dreams can and do come true. If you open your mind to what could be and manifest your purpose—incredible things are possible.

And science proves it.

Let's start from the beginning. While babies don't have a conscious, articulated sense of purpose like adults, they do have drives and motivations. These forces propel them into exploration of the world around them, into seeking connection with their caregivers and then other humans—that all-important attachment they need, that we talked about before. Their needs, desires, and then curiosity push them to develop skills they need to survive. The actions and thought processes being laid down in infanthood are precursors to the development of a more complex sense of purpose later in life. You could say that babies have *proto-purposes* or *pre-purposes* that set the stage for later development. Then, even in very young children, we see the beginnings of a recognizable sense of purpose. Kids have a strong desire to build things, to help friends, to care for animals—and to explore how their actions have an impact on the world that surrounds them. We see them develop restraint, self-control, a sense of altruism. As they grow up, teenagers then start to explore their values, interests, and potential roles in society. They find purpose in causes, in talents they want to develop, in allegiances to certain groups (such as sports teams, bands, or public figures); they explore relationships that open entirely new dimensions of emotion.

In adulthood, it seems we are supposed to have our purpose figured out. As we progress through our education, we choose and pursue a path of study. We take a job that is meant to evolve into a career. We enter committed relationships, start families, settle in communities. We can carry with us a calling from early on in life that leads us to a sense of purpose as we do so, some in our professional lives. Others of us feel a sense of purpose in raising children, practicing our faith, or giving of our time and resources to others. But sometimes, it feels as if things happen in a way that we don't expect. We make a decision that leads us down a different path, and several forks in the road later, we feel lost. That happened to me.

Science has tried to measure a sense of purpose, and as this is something deeply personal and subjective, it presents a real challenge for scientists and medical professionals. It's not like taking a person's temperature or measuring their blood pressure. Researchers have had to get creative to try to find as many empirical ways as possible to assess it. One common approach is to use questionnaires, where the answers correlate to scales that give self-reported measures of mental health and well-being, as we discussed in the last chapter about hope. For our purpose, there are metrics such as the Purpose in Life test, developed in 1964 to measure one's sense of perceived purpose or meaning in life. The test is based on Holocaust survivor and psychologist Viktor Frankl's concepts, developed in his multimillion-copy bestselling book, *Man's Search for Meaning*. The respondent is asked to rank how strongly they agree or disagree with a number of statements, and a score is tallied that shows the strength of a person's sense of meaning or purpose. Here are a few of the statements:

- Life seems to me: completely routine / always exciting.
- In life I have: no goals or aims / clear goals and aims.
- My personal existence is: utterly meaningless, without purpose / purposeful and meaningful.
- Every day is: exactly the same / constantly new and different.
- If I could choose, I would: prefer to never have been born / want nine more lives just like this one.
- If I should die today, I'd feel that my life has been: completely worthless / very worthwhile.
- In thinking of my life, I: often wonder why I exist / always see reasons for being here.

A more recent test to measure purpose is the Sense of Purpose Scale, developed in 2017 and described in the journal *Applied Developmental Science*. The authors note the need "to have a clear conceptualization and a psychometrically sound measurement of this construct" and their intent "to design, develop, and test validity and reliability of a multidimensional measure of purpose." Their scale measures results based on responses to questions, which are then grouped into categories including altruistic purpose, awareness of purpose, awakening to purpose, presence of meaning, search for meaning, compassion, extrinsic religion, and social desirability. The assessment is weighted in response to how strongly the test taker agrees with statements including:

- I have begun to contemplate what I ultimately wish to achieve.
- I am striving to make a positive difference in society.
- I am in the process of formulating my long-term goals.
- My life's purpose has nothing to do with common good.
- My current aims match with my future aspirations.
- My current activities have helped me to develop clear aims.
- I seek to learn so that I can help others.
- I have started thinking about what I truly want to achieve.
- I have often volunteered to contribute to the welfare of others.
- I feel aimless.

Some scales designed to measure overall psychological well-being also include subscales that touch on purpose that are helpful; for instance, the Ryff Inventory, developed by psychologist Carol D. Ryff in 1989, looks at six aspects of well-being and happiness: autonomy, environmental mastery, personal growth, positive relations with others, purpose in life, and self-acceptance.

Beyond questionnaires, researchers sometimes turn to interviews to explore sense of purpose with subjects in a more conversational way. This allows for less structured, open-ended questions that let people share their stories in their own way. Researchers have to then analyze these narratives that people construct about their lives, looking for recurring themes related to purpose and direction.

Researchers look not only at what people say they believe, but how they behave. Do people set meaningful goals and work toward them? Are they involved in volunteer work or civic engagement? These actions offer clues about an individual's sense of purpose.

The challenge is that purpose is so personal. What gives one person meaning might be entirely different for someone else. Cultural context plays a role, too, shaping how people understand and express what they see as meaningful in life.

What appears consistent, though, is that having a sense of purpose, however one defines it internally, has a direct impact on your health. A 2021 edition of the medical journal *Circulation*, published by the American Heart Association, cited several fascinating studies, noting:

> Adults with a greater sense of purpose have more favorable lifestyle and cardiovascular risk factors such as less smoking, more physical activity, less alcohol and substance abuse, and better glucose control. A greater sense of purpose in life has been associated with better cardiovascular health, longevity, and reduced risk of CVD, including decreased risk of both MI [myocardial infarction] and stroke. Older adults who have a greater sense of purpose in life also had a lower risk of mortality, even after accounting for depression, disability, and other comorbidities.

A 2016 meta-analysis published in the journal *Psychosomatic Medicine* took a look at studies done with 136,265 participants. Findings showed "significant association between having a higher purpose in life and reduced all-cause mortality and cardiovascular events."

How is this possible? Where is all of this coming from? Well, perhaps unsurprisingly, a lot of it connects back to stress. People with a strong sense of purpose tend to experience less intense bodily responses to stress. They have a lower emotional reactivity in general, meaning for instance that their heart rate and blood pressure don't spike as dramatically in challenging situations. This keeps their systems more regulated. As noted in a 2018 study called "Sense of Purpose Moderates the Associations Between Daily Stressors and Daily Well-Being," published in *The Annals of Behavioral Medicine*, "research suggests that a higher sense of purpose is associated with lower levels of perceived stress and reduced cortisol reactivity and output."

People with a sense of purpose are not as prone to suffer from chronic stress, meaning they are also less likely to have chronic inflammation—which is in turn linked to numerous chronic diseases including some neurodegenerative conditions, heart disease, and diabetes. Studies have shown that people with a sense of purpose tend to have lower levels of inflammatory markers in their blood. There are some indicators that people with a sense of purpose also have more robust immune systems; for instance, they may have enhanced production of antibodies that fight off infections. Having a sense of purpose might even influence our epigenetics, affecting how our genes are turned on or off, which in turn fundamentally impacts our health and resilience. At the cellular level, telomere length is predictive of how the body reacts to aging and disease. Telomeres are protective caps on the ends of chromosomes, and shorter telomeres are associated with aging and disease. Though the results are inconclusive so far, some research suggests that purpose can help maintain telomere length, helping cells stay healthier, longer.

Pursue Your Purpose

As mentioned in the *Circulation* study, there are also lifestyle factors associated with a sense of purpose that significantly impact health. People take better care of their bodies when they feel their lives have meaning and value—leading them to better lifestyle choices on exercise and diet. Purpose can also discourage risky behaviors, self-destructive coping mechanisms such as excessive alcohol consumption or drug use. Basically, people with purpose feel they have more of a reason to take care of themselves, which, as we have seen, contributes to their ability to mount a Resilience Response.

As I mentioned earlier, some are fortunate enough to feel a sense of purpose emerge naturally in their lives. It's not uncommon to hear a pastor, doctor, or social worker talk about feeling called to their work from a young age. But for others, a sense of purpose emerges from something incredibly unfortunate and out of the blue. I'll never forget working on gun-safety issues for a segment on CBS, where we were making the case that this issue represents a national health emergency. I spoke with a trauma surgeon who has treated young gunshot victims and with three parents of children who had been killed by unsecured firearms. One of the moms, Gwendolyn La Croix, became a pediatric psychiatric nurse practitioner and a leader in the anti-gun-violence advocacy group Moms Demand Action after she lost her son Jonah. Another mom, Kristin Song, successfully lobbied for a state law called Ethan's Law, strengthening requirements for safe storage of firearms in homes, and is pushing for a federal version. Kristin had no idea why her son, Ethan, was at the hospital when she got the call. She explained, "Waiting for the ER doctor to come in, we had no idea Ethan had been shot. I thought he had gotten hit by a car." Ethan had accidentally shot and killed himself at his friend's house after the two of them posted pictures on social media showing them goofing around, holding a gun. "Eight children a day are dying because they've gained access to a gun," Song told me in an interview. Thirty states and the District of Columbia have now passed child-access-prevention laws like Ethan's Law.

There are countless other stories of parents of children with diseases putting aside their lives to crusade for a cure, and quieter stories of people devoting themselves to caregiving for family members who have disabilities or degenerative conditions.

For others still, finding their purpose doesn't necessarily happen early in life or like a bolt from the blue. For some people it's more like planting a tree: It takes time, effort, and consistent nurturing—especially at first. It may take years before your efforts bear fruit. One of the first steps is looking inward, digging deep to understand your values. What principles guide your decisions? What kind of person do you aspire to be? What mark do you want to leave on the world? Ask yourself these questions and dig deep to find the answers.

If you want to take another route, take time to consider and explore your passions. What ignites your curiosity? What activities make you lose track of time? Sometimes revisiting things you enjoyed as a child can spark that same sense of wonder and enjoyment. It's also great to encourage yourself to try new things, too; sometimes there's a sport, hobby, or artistic pursuit you have been curious about for years but have perhaps been too nervous to try. Once you get going, look for activities that fully absorb you and leave you feeling energized and fulfilled.

Or maybe you'd like to try activities that lead to meaningful engagement with others. Think about how you can contribute to something bigger than yourself, whether it's volunteering, taking part in some kind of group activity in your community, or simply offering a helping hand to those around you in an immediate and daily way. Consider how you can use your unique skills and talents—or just your natural human empathy—to make a positive difference. Connecting with others is essential, as we've discussed. Strong relationships with family, friends, and community members provide a sense of belonging and support. And remember the power of giving and receiving support; it can be a profound source of meaning in and of itself.

There are many professions devoted to the care and support of others, including teaching, social work, childcare, and countless others. The tangible, direct, and fundamental way that the practice of medicine supports others is the biggest reason I was drawn to the field. But even when we pursue a career that aligns with our deepest sense of purpose, there will be challenges. I certainly found that to be true in my experience as a doctor. It helps to remember that core purpose when times get hard. Becoming a healthcare provider means committing to a life of giving to others: giving time, mental and physical energy, and in some cases even sacrificing one's own safety and health to keep others alive and healthy. Healthcare workers walk in that liminal space between joy and success and suffering, pain, and death. That space can be wonderful but also draining.

When you are helping patients day in and day out—some of whom will thrive, but others who won't—it's hard not to feel the weight of your practice. I've been in medicine for over twenty years and one of the issues that comes up time and time again among my colleagues and peers is burnout. The World Health Organization describes burnout as "an occupational phenomenon," identified by the following characteristics: "feelings of energy depletion or exhaustion; increased mental distance from one's job, or feelings of negativism or cynicism related to one's job; and reduced professional efficacy." The last five years have been particularly and extraordinarily challenging in healthcare. COVID was a rough time to be a doctor or nurse. After New Yorkers stopped banging on pots and pans every night, after the acute period of the pandemic ended, variants kept popping up like whack-a-mole, and the revolutionary and lifesaving vaccines were quickly politicized. And yet, frontline workers continued to put the well-being of their patients above their own. Researchers affiliated with the Mayo Clinic, the Stanford University School of Medicine, the University of Colorado School of Medicine, and the American Medical Association conducted a study, published in *Mayo Clinic Proceedings*, that found that as compared to 38.2 percent in 2020, 62.8 percent of physicians surveyed experienced at least one characteristic related to burnout by the end of 2021.

Dennis Charney, the biological psychiatrist with the NIH I mentioned in the first chapter of this book, was on the ground during the pandemic and saw this firsthand. When I interviewed him in the aftermath of 2020, he said, "On one hand, it was an unprecedented year in terms of the level of stress that our faculty and staff were under. On the other hand, the bravery and the courage that our frontline healthcare workers, nurses, doctors, respiratory therapists, have been under—I've never seen it like this. The challenge has been enormous, but response has been terrific."

I asked him to explain a bit more about how he saw doctors and nurses and hospital staff dig deep to find the resilience they needed to keep coming to work each day. What he told me directly linked to a sense of purpose: "The frontline workers [experienced] a sense of fear for their own health and the health of their family when they went home. . . . On the other hand, and this was remarkable, the meaning that they attributed to their job went up enormously. They felt, you know, 'This is what I was trained for. I have an obligation to work on the front line and work to save lives.' . . . What surprised me was the courage and bravery and the enhanced sense of meaning. . . . Those of us who study resilience say ordinary people can do extraordinary things. And that's what we saw in the height of the pandemic." He continued, "When I asked them, 'How are you handling this?', they would say, 'Well, this is why I went into healthcare.' . . . The stress was unbelievable and unrelenting. Day after day after day working extraordinary hours. And also having to be redeployed from the area that you were trained in, to now take care of COVID patients."

He described how they created a resilience program at Mount Sinai in the spring of 2020, a center for stress, resilience, and personal growth that offered free assessment and care to frontline healthcare workers. He told me, "You know, our motto is 'We take care of our own.' I think it was one of the first [centers like this] in the country. And our staff, our leadership, have gone around the country talking to other healthcare systems about what we did." Even though the pandemic is over, the center is still open and will remain so.

Because the need remains. According to Definitive Healthcare, 145,213 healthcare professionals left the industry between 2021 and 2022. That number includes almost 35,000 nurse practitioners and roughly 71,000 physicians. And these mass departures only made the burnout problem worse. As hospitals became more and more short-staffed, the medical professionals who did stick around felt even greater pressure, leading to further departures. Various publications by the Association of American Medical Colleges have reported that physician demand will far overwhelm supply by 2033. Furthermore, the US Department of Health has projected that by this year, roughly forty-five thousand to ninety thousand providers will be faced with "poor working conditions and high levels of stress." The problem is so dire that much as he did with social isolation, Dr. Vivek Murthy, the surgeon general under President Biden, put out an advisory noting the extreme importance of medical-worker burnout.

The Healing Power of Resilience

Burnout isn't inevitable. There are a lot of different ways of combating it, including investing in positive work environments and providing support to providers. But to me, the most important tool in this fight is purpose. The research bears this out, too. In a 2022 survey of 127 doctors from seventy different hospitals, researchers found that while doctors who work at both profit-driven and purpose-driven hospitals can be satisfied in their jobs, only doctors at the latter find them to be meaningful. When things get tough and it's hard to see the light at the end of the tunnel, it's helpful to have a strong sense of purpose that keeps you going. It also helps to think about your purpose more holistically: To live a purposeful life doesn't only mean doing your best work for others in your professional setting, but also remembering your sense of purpose as a family member, friend, sibling, partner, and source of support to others in your life.

One of the most gripping stories I've ever heard of a doctor with a true sense of purpose is that of Dr. Joseph Sakran. A trauma surgeon at Johns Hopkins Hospital in a tough corner of downtown Baltimore, Sakran has seen more than his fair share of bullet wounds. His path into medicine began when he was almost fatally shot in the throat as a teenager, the unintended victim of gang violence. The vascular surgeon who treated him was only two years out of training and had to think and work fast to save Sakran's life. The surgeon, Dr. Robert Ahmed, took a vein from Sakran's leg to replace the torn vessel in his neck, and thankfully it worked. Sakran's recovery was long and arduous, but it was also something of a miracle. Then, once he left the hospital and resumed his life, Sakran did what most people don't: He went back into the hospital, again and again. As a college student attending school nearby, he signed up to volunteer in that same hospital's emergency department. Dr. Ahmed, the surgeon who saved his life, remembers attending to a patient when he saw Sakran. "I said, 'Joe, what the hell are you doing here?' Most trauma survivors stay well away." Sakran said he wanted to prove to the doctor that what he did, what his team did, was not a waste. Sakran told him, "I may not look as good as you with my scars. But, you know, I got the second chance." With that second chance Sakran not only pursued a career as a trauma surgeon but also as an outspoken advocate against gun violence. In November 2018, the NRA fired off a tweet warning "self-important anti-gun doctors to stay in their lane." The message went viral, fueling more than twenty-one thousand responses and the ire of doctors across the United States. When Sakran saw the NRA's message, he felt a wave of disbelief—and then just rage. "As a Trauma Surgeon and survivor of #GunViolence I cannot believe the audacity of the @NRA. . . . Where are you when I'm having to tell all those families their loved one has died?"

Sakran decided to do something productive with his anger and founded an online community called This Is Our Lane. Thousands of doctors started posting stories and pictures: graphic, tragic, gruesome, heartbreaking words and images. Sakran now not only calls himself a doctor but an advocate, and his efforts have paid off. He was instrumental in helping to establish the first White House Office of Gun Violence Prevention in September 2023.

Clearly Sakran feels fueled by a deep sense of purpose in his practice of medicine. Carol Horowitz, a professor of population health science and policy and professor of medicine at the Icahn School of Medicine at Mt. Sinai, saw so clearly that job satisfaction in medicine was tied to meaningfulness that she and her fellow researchers sought to drill down on what makes these jobs meaningful in the first place. Over six years in the early to mid-nineties, Horowitz and her coauthors conducted workshops at annual meetings of the Society of General Internal Medicine and the American College of Physicians and asked participants to tell them about experiences they found meaningful. Ultimately, the researchers developed themes from these stories, such as doctor-patient intimacy and the ability to make a difference in a patient's life. And furthermore, those who participated in these workshops found that sharing these stories was fulfilling in itself—a conclusion that the researchers suggested might be helpful in the medical practice in general.

Sharing these stories echoes a conclusion that came out of the surgeon general's advisory on burnout. One of its chief recommendations was to "recognize social connection and community as a core value of the health care system." The advisory emphasized that strengthening the bonds both within the medical community and the community around it would enhance job satisfaction for medical workers.

In its own recommendations, the American Medical Association developed a Physician Well-Being Program. One of this program's explicit goals is to "promote joy, meaning, and purpose to the practice of medicine," grounded in the belief that doing so would stave off the epidemic of medical workers exiting the professional. The AMA even established something called the Joy in Medicine program, which is intended to, as the name suggests, promote well-being among staffs at health systems that employ over seventy-five physicians. For example, the AMA recommends that these institutions establish leadership roles specifically responsible for physician happiness.

Most doctors I know entered the profession to help people—and for me, it's intuitive that focusing on that purpose, while trying to improve other aspects of our work environment, will help quell its problems. For years now, the AMA has published a series of first-person narratives called "The Moment I Knew Medicine Was My Calling." In these interviews, doctors talk about what personally brings them meaning in their respective practices. Take Dr. Michael S. Sinha, a postdoctoral fellow at

Brigham and Women's Hospital in Boston. When asked about the most rewarding part of his job, he explained, "People are extremely candid with their physicians, and there's no better way to respect that vulnerability than to listen." Dr. Fatima Cody Stanford, an obesity-medicine physician at Massachusetts General Hospital in Boston, took it a step farther. She explains, "In medical school, I was often told that I should minimize my expectations, since striving for challenging goals would only lead to disappointment. Thus, I chose the alternate pathway, and I continue to strive for the highest heights possible. I've never looked back."

Doctors and nurses aren't the only people who keep on going because they are motivated by a sense of purpose. Throughout this book, I've written about people who worked hard to strengthen their resilience and, at the heart of each of these examples, were the stories of how they found their purpose.

Recall the case of BJ Miller, who found his purpose as a palliative caregiver after a near-fatal accident, or Gabby Giffords, who has found her purpose—and her voice—advocating for aphasia patients as well as tirelessly working to end gun violence. When I think about purpose, I also think a lot about a woman named Sonja Wasden, whom I interviewed for CBS News in November 2020. Sonja suffers from bipolar disorder and is a suicide survivor. She and her daughter cowrote a book about their journey called *An Impossible Life* and have traveled across the country speaking and giving copies away to libraries to share hope with others who struggle with their mental health.

Throughout her ongoing struggle with mental illness, Wasden has had to call upon her resilience to keep going—which is bolstered by the support of her loving family, by taking care of herself through regular visits with medical professionals, and by the sense of purpose she finds in helping others by sharing her experiences and talking openly about mental health.

The Healing Power of Resilience

She told me, "I would say that you have to radically accept some things in your life . . . as humans that we sometimes fight against, some of the trials or difficulties that we have. But I think once we're able to radically accept and say, 'It is what it is,' and then to embrace it and bring it into your life and say, 'I can live with this,' and you figure out a way to do it."

Sonja went on to say, "I have a beautiful life now. My marriage of twenty-seven years is going strong. I have good relationships with all my children. I don't stay in bed all day anymore. I am out participating in life and fully engaged. Yes, I have a mental illness. And, yes, I have moments of pain and anxiety and difficulty. It's a lifelong illness that I have to manage. But I can have a life worth living, too." I love the idea that what feels like an impossible life can become one that feels like a life worth living—and a beautiful one at that. Sonja's resilience has allowed her to pursue her purpose: "There is something almost beautiful that happens [when you] release yourself. Instead of trying to control it, you let go and accept it and invite it into your life and embrace it. . . . Your eyes have been opened to other people's suffering and how you can lift [them]."

Finding one's purpose can be quiet and personal, too. As Gus's example from the last chapter shows us, uncovering your purpose can be private, such as realizing you'll find more meaning and more fulfillment in showing up for your grandchildren's baseball games and cooking classes than winning a big case in court. Recently something special arrived at my office that reminded me of this. It was a beautiful card from one of my patients. On the cover was a piece of artwork he had painted himself, and inside was a perfect message, a quote by noted psychiatrist and author David Viscott: "The purpose of life is to discover your gift. The work of life is to develop it. The meaning of life is to give your gift away."

Here is my gift to you: these words, this book. I hope it helps you to build your resilience and enjoy to the utmost the beautiful life you have.

Epilogue

Throughout this book, I've talked about treating patients as whole people, and I've been sharing my experiences as a doctor and a health journalist, but also as a college student and a daughter, wife, and mother. No surprise, I am a whole person, too. Yes, I love studying the heart and keeping up with the latest medical advances, and learning about the practice of medicine from my patients and from my health reporting. I also love movies and music. I love to travel, especially to Italy.

In 1997, the year I graduated from Stanford, a movie was released called *La vita è bella*. Set in my favorite place in the world—Tuscany, Italy—Roberto Benigni's film is about war, family, love, optimism, hope, and the strength of the human soul to overcome darkness and tragedy. The film moved me then, and I realize now it was because it was all about resilience and the innate capacity of humans to persevere through adversity and to be a light for others. It is also a reminder that despite what happens to us, life is beautiful.

I look around at my patients, the stories of people I have interviewed for the news, my family and friends, and I see a sea of infinite resilience.

Epilogue

Resilience is a part of who we are—always there inside us, to build on throughout our lives. When the waves come and your world is rocked by difficulty, be it in your health or something else, remember you are stronger than you think. In those moments, bounce forward.

As we look ahead to where our resilience can take us on our journey, I believe it's also important to remember to appreciate and have gratitude for where we are and what we have in the present moment. I often think about the lyrics of Josh Groban's song "Granted," released in 2018. Music has always been a way to calm my soul, and this song has been special for me. Josh Groban said in an interview the song "is about not taking anything for granted. It is also about granting yourself the permission to take the leap when you don't think you can . . . to help people see that there is a light, they can follow that light and they can do great things in the world, they can do great things for themselves." I won't quote the song at length here, but I encourage you to listen to it.

May this book be a guide; a home you can always come back to; a reminder to never take a single breath for granted; a resource that will lift you up and inspire you to believe that no matter what you are facing, you can enjoy your life, even if a new baseline is required.

Acknowledgments

Writing this book has been a labor of love and would not have been possible without the love and support of so many people along the way. The road to publishing my first book has been shaped by all of you, and I can't ever thank you enough.

First I have to thank Susan Zirinsky for pointing S&S in my direction and believing there was a book inside my brain. Thank you to my brilliant editor Emily Graff, who from day one as my new editor has been there with her unwavering optimism, belief, and help in making sure this book was everything it should be and more. Thank you, Emily, for cheering me on and for being an incredible rock of support. It has been a privilege to work with you. Thank you to Leah Miller, my first editor at S&S, Richard Rhorer, Katie McClimon, the art/design group, and the whole team at Simon & Schuster who have believed in this book from the beginning and have patiently allowed it to evolve and take flight. Shannon O'Neill and Emily Heckman brought this vision to life. Thank you, Shannon and Emily, for understanding me and my dream and navigating this road to create something truly remarkable. I loved

Acknowledgments

working with you and your spirit and dedication to this book are infused in each page. I am grateful to Ariel Doctoroff, who also gave her time, patience, and assistance in making sure every detail was correct. Thank you as well to my literary agent Gail Ross and my media agent Rachel Adler for always looking out for me in every way. I have to extend thanks to my very first media agent Janet Pawson, who believed in my ability and dream of working in television.

CBS News was my first home where I learned to spread my wings as a journalist. I am grateful to my special producers at CBS who helped me tell stories many of which became part of this book and were essential in my evolution as a medical correspondent. Thank you Susie Schackman, Leigh Ann Winick, Heather Won Tesoriero, Natasha Singh, Sarah Longden, and Andrew Merlis for being some of the best producers ever. I am also thankful for my wonderful medical team of producers at ABC News including Eric Strauss, Jessica Yankelunas, Sony Salzman, Youri Benadjaoud, Liz Neporent, Greg Tufaro, and Cathy Becker for helping me continue to do the work I love and for your constant support.

Today I am blessed to work with Dr. Stacey Rosen, Dr. Jennifer Mieres, Dr. Jeff Kuvin, and Dr. Varinder Singh and my wonderful office manager Sally Ng at Northwell Health, who have supported my dual career path and have been in my corner each step of the way.

The book has also been cultivated by my experience with my patients. I thank my patients for the honor of caring for them, for their vulnerability, for sharing their hearts and souls with me, and for their wisdom, humor, and teaching.

Getting to this point in my career would not have been possible without the support of the many physicians who have believed in me along the way. Thank you to Dr. Astrid Heger for being a beacon of hope to so many and for sharing your gift with me. I promise, Astrid, to always

Acknowledgments

make medicine personal. Thank you to Dr. Marshall Wolf and Dr. Joel Katz at the Brigham and Women's Hospital, who believed in my pursuit of an alternate career in medical journalism and fostered a culture where residents who trained under them could soar. One of the greatest gifts of my residency was that it brought me my incredible group of female best friends and fellow doctors: Nazleen, Jenn, Sandra, Risha, Kate, Julie, Melissa, Lynn, Jen. Your friendship, love, and laughter are so precious to me, and I cherish you all so much. You helped me survive medical training and life beyond. Thank you to Dr. Erica Jones, who fought for me to be able to leave my cardiology fellowship one day a week in my final year of cardiology training to participate in an NBC internship, which was the first step in my media career. Thanks to Roxanne Garcia Bell and Jane Derenowski at NBC News, who gave me the unique opportunity to learn about the inner workings of medical journalism during my internship. My initial steps in media were also supported by Brooks Lancaster, who helped me get my first spot on a national morning show. Thanks as well to Nancy Brown at the American Heart Association for always raising up my work and efforts. Thank you, Alison Hilton, for being such a beautiful friend and helping me always find my way with your love and compassion and kindness. Thank you, Anjelica, Jerry, Deacon Vic, Anne, and all the other angels who have gently guided me along the way. For me spirituality has been a big part of my journey, and I also must thank my special saint, Padre Pio, for always watching over me and shining a light on my path to comfort me and show me the way.

Finally, family has always been the foundation and most important part of my life. To my family, I love you all so very much. Mom and Dad, thank you for all you sacrificed, all you taught me, and for all your endless love, support, and belief in me. Thank you to my brother Karr and his family for their love and for always rooting for me. Thank you

Acknowledgments

Barbara, Carl, Ryan, Anne, and Chris, for always being there for me with your love and support. The best part of my life began when I met my husband, David. David has been a constant support of my work and my dreams from the beginning. He has taught me so much about life and love and so much more. Thank you, Dave, for everything, and I'm so grateful to be by your side in this journey and for all your encouragement and love. I love you forever and always. My two incredibly special daughters, Siena and Layla, have been in my mind each and every step of the way writing this book. I know life will bring you challenges, and I hope this book can be a guide for you as you make your way in the world. I want this book to be a reminder that you can ride the waves, you can always find the sunshine, and that love is all around you. Thank you, Siena and Layla, for your love, for making me smile, and for being the brilliant stars in my sky.

Notes

Introduction

xiii *Cardiovascular disease kills more*; Olga Khavjou et al., "Projections of Cardiovascular Disease Prevalence and Costs: 2015–2035," Technical Report, RTI International, October 2016, https://www.heart.org/en/-/media/Files/Get-Involved/Advocacy/Burden-Report-Technical-Report.pdf.

Chapter 1: The Origins of the Resilience Response

6 *For instance, there is evidence that a positive mindset*: S. J. Schleifer and S. E. Keller, "The Influence of Psychological Factors on Immunity," *Dialogues in Clinical Neuroscience* 2, no. 2 (2000): 99–108.

6 *Exercising regularly can improve mental well-being for all of us*: Na Li et al., "The Association Between Physical Exercise Behavior and Psychological Resilience of Teenagers: An Examination of the Chain Mediating Effect," *Scientific Reports* 14, no. 1 (April 23, 2024), https://doi.org/10.1038/s41598-024-60038-1.

7 *In the 1950s, psychologist and researcher Abraham Maslow*: Roy José DeCarvalho, "The Growth Hypothesis in Psychology: The Humanistic Psychology of Abraham Maslow and Carl Rogers" (San Francisco: EM Text, 1991), https://cir.nii.ac.jp/crid/1130282269014784256.

8 *"not necessarily impervious[ness] to stress"*: Norman Garmezy, "Resiliency and Vulnerability to Adverse Developmental Outcomes Associated with Poverty," *American Behavioral Scientist* 34, no. 4 (March 1, 1991): 416–30, https://doi.org/10.1177/0002764291034004003.

8 *He made a career studying*: Ibid.

8 *Take, for example, a 2020 study*: Bruce J. Ellis et al., "Hidden Talents in Harsh Environments," *Development and Psychopathology* 34, no. 1 (July 16, 2020): 95–113, https://doi.org/10.1017/s0954579420000887.

9 *In another fascinating study across the Atlantic*: Michael Rutter, "Developmental Catch-Up, and Deficit, Following Adoption After Severe Global Early

Notes

Privation," *Journal of Child Psychology and Psychiatry* 39, no. 4 (May 1, 1998): 465–76, https://doi.org/10.1111/1469-7610.00343.

9 *He compared Romanian children*: Ibid.

10 *Werner, based on her studies of children*: Emmy E. Werner and Ruth S. Smith, *Overcoming the Odds* (Ithaca, NY: Cornell University Press, 1992), https://doi.org/10.7591/9781501711992.

10 *"the ability to bend but not break"*: Steven M. Southwick et al., "Resilience Definitions, Theory, and Challenges: Interdisciplinary Perspectives," *European Journal of Psychotraumatology* 5, no. 1 (October 1, 2024), https://doi.org/10.3402/ejpt.v5.25338.

10 *In the mid-1990s*: R. G. Tedeschi and L. G. Calhoun, "The Posttraumatic Growth Inventory: Measuring the Positive Legacy of Trauma," *Journal of Traumatic Stress* 9, no. 3 (July 1996), https://doi.org/10.1002/jts.2490090305.

10 *"People develop new understandings"*: Lorna Collier, "Growth After Trauma: Why Are Some People More Resilient Than Others—and Can It Be Taught?," *Monitor on Psychology* 47, no. 10 (November 2016), https://www.apa.org/monitor/2016/11/growth-trauma.

11 *Tedeschi and Calhoun went on to create*: Tedeschi and Calhoun, "Posttraumatic Growth Inventory."

11 *His theory of resilience*: George A. Bonanno et al., "Loss and Human Resilience," *Applied and Preventative Psychology* 10, no. 3 (Summer 2001), https://doi.org/10.1016/S0962-1849(01)80014-7.

11 *His discovery highlighted*: George A. Bonanno et al., "Resilience to Loss and Potential Trauma," *Annual Review of Clinical Psychology* 7 (2011), https://doi.org/10.1146/annurev-clinpsy-032210-104526.

11 *The factors that bolster*: Isaac R. Galatzer-Levy et al., "Trajectories of Resilience and Dysfunction Following Potential Trauma: A Review and Statistical Evaluation," *Clinical Psychology Review* 63 (2018), https://doi.org/10.1016/j.cpr.2018.05.008.

11 *In essence, we all possess the ability*: Katharina Schultebraucks et al., "Discriminating Heterogeneous Trajectories of Resilience and Depression After Major Life Stressors Using Polygenic Scores," *JAMA Psychiatry* 78, no. 7 (July 2021), https://doi.org/10.1001/jamapsychiatry.2021.0228.

12 *Based on what he's learned so far*: George A. Bonanno, "The Resilience Paradox," *European Journal of Psychotraumatology* 12, no. 1 (June 30, 2021), https://doi.org/10.1080/20008198.2021.1942642.

12 *Picking up on the work of Tedeschi and Calhoun and others*: Andrew Joseph, "As a Scientist, He Studied Trauma Victims. Then He Became One," *STAT*, September 21, 2017, https://www.statnews.com/2017/09/21/resilience-trauma-research/.

12 *Charney called his findings the 10 Essential Principles of Resilience*: Dennis Charney, "The Resilience Prescription," Icahn School of Medicine at Mount Sinai, https://

Notes

icahn.mssm.edu/files/ISMMS/Assets/Files/Resilience-Prescription-Promotion.pdf.

16 *And the medical experiences of women and minorities*: Maggie Fox, "Sex Matters: Medical Research Overlooks Women," *Fuller Project*, November 20, 2023, https://fullerproject.org/story/sex-matters-medical-research-overlooks-women/.

16 *For example, a study published in the* Journal of the American Heart Association: Laura Williamson, "The Slowly Evolving Truth About Heart Disease and Women," American Heart Association, February 9, 2024, https://www.heart.org/en/news/2024/02/09/the-slowly-evolving-truth-about-heart-disease-and-women.

16 *Another study, published in* JAMA Network Open: Chirag M. Vyas et al., "Association of Race and Ethnicity with Late-Life Depression Severity, Symptom Burden, and Care," *JAMA Network Open* 3, no. 3 (March 26, 2020), https://www.doi.org/10.1001/jamanetworkopen.2020.1606.

Chapter 2: Why Stress Is the Heart of the Matter

17 *Every thirty-four seconds*: "Heart Disease Facts," Centers for Disease Control, October 24, 2024, https://www.cdc.gov/heart-disease/data-research/facts-stats/index.html.

18 *"most forms of psychological distress"*: Glenn N. Levine et al., "Psychological Health, Well-Being, and the Mind-Heart-Body Connection: A Scientific Statement from the American Heart Association," *Circulation* 143, no. 10 (January 25, 2021), https://doi.org/10.1161/CIR.0000000000000947.

21 *"A zebra's stress response kicks in"*: Robert M. Sapolsky, *Why Zebras Don't Get Ulcers* (New York: Holt Paperbacks, 2004).

22 *Chronic stress also leads to chronic high blood pressure*: Ahmed Tawakol et al., "Relation Between Resting Amygdalar Activity and Cardiovascular Events: A Longitudinal and Cohort Study," *Lancet* 389, no. 10071 (February 25, 2017): 834–45, https://doi.org/10.1016/S0140-6736(16)31714-7.

24 *Then, when we encounter a stressful situation*: Firdaus S. Dhabhar, "Effects of Stress on Immune Function: The Good, the Bad, and the Beautiful," *Immunologic Research* 58 (May 2014): 193–210, https://doi.org/10.1007/s12026-014-8517-0.

25 *we may find our diet becomes overreliant on sugars and carbs*: Garvan Institute of Medical Research, "How Chronic Stress Drives the Brain to Crave Comfort Food," *ScienceDaily*, June 8, 2023, https://www.sciencedaily.com/releases/2023/06/230608120905.htm.

25 *However, fewer than 7 percent of these people*: "How Common Is PTSD in Veterans?," National Center for PTSD, US Department of Veterans Affairs, https://www.ptsd.va.gov/understand/common/common_veterans.asp.

25 *The majority of people who experience*: Jonathan E. Sherin and Charles B. Nemeroff, "Post-Traumatic Stress Disorder: The Neurobiological Impact of Psychological Trauma," *Dialogues in Clinical Neuroscience* 13, no. 3 (2011): 263–78, https://doi.org/10.31887/DCNS.2011.13.2/jsherin.

Notes

26 *most of us can experience and process highly traumatic events*: George A. Bonanno, *The End of Trauma: How the New Science of Resilience Is Changing How We Think About PTSD* (New York: Hachette, 2021).

26 *fully 65 percent of people who went through these difficult experiences*: George A. Bonanno et al., "Psychological Resilience After Disaster: New York in the Aftermath of the September 11th Terrorist Attack," *Psychological Science* 17, no. 3 (March 2006): 181–86, https://doi.org/10.1111/j.1467-9280.2006.01682.x.

27 *the "resilience paradox"*: George A. Bonanno, "The Resilience Paradox," *European Journal of Psychotraumatology* 12, no. 1 (June 2021), https://doi.org/10.1080/20008198.2021.1942642.

27 *For instance, several studies have looked at the hippocampus*: Mikael Rubin et al., "Greater Hippocampal Volume Is Associated with PTSD Treatment Response," *Psychiatry Research: Neuroimaging* 252 (June 30, 2016): 36–39, https://doi.org/10.1016/j.pscychresns.2016.05.001.

28 *It would make sense, then, that early interventions*: J. P. Hayes, M. B. VanElzakker, and L. M. Shin, "Effects of Cognitive Behavioral Therapy on Hippocampal Volume in Posttraumatic Stress Disorder: A Meta-Analysis," *Journal of Psychiatric Research* 46, no. 10 (2012): 1331–37.

28 *The Mount Sinai program and others like it*: "WTC Health Program History," Centers for Disease Control, cdc.gov, March 7, 2025, https://www.cdc.gov/wtc/history.html.

29 *Research has shown that prior exposure to trauma*: Sabra S. Inslicht, "Family Psychiatric History, Peritraumatic Reactivity, and Posttraumatic Stress Symptoms: A Prospective Study of Policy," *Journal of Psychiatric Research* 44, no. 1 (January 2010): 22–31, https://doi.org/10.1016/j.jpsychires.2009.05.011.

29 *Studies also show that approximately one-third*: Lynn M. Almli et al., "Genetic Approaches to Understanding Post-Traumatic Stress Disorder," *International Journal of Neuropsychopharmacology* 17, no. 2 (February 2014): 355–70, https://doi.org/10.1017/S1461145713001090.

30 *The US government's Office of Disease Prevention and Health Promotion (ODPHP) recommends*: *Physical Activity Guidelines for Americans*, 2nd ed., US Department of Health and Human Services, 2018, https://odphp.health.gov/sites/default/files/2019-09/Physical_Activity_Guidelines_2nd_edition.pdf.

30 *Those who exceeded these guidelines*: "New Study Finds Lowest Risk of Death Was Among Adults Who Exercised 150–600 Minutes/Week," *Circulation Journal Report*, July 25, 2022, https://newsroom.heart.org/news/new-study-finds-lowest-risk-of-death-was-among-adults-who-exercised-150-600-minutesweek.

34 *Over the fifty years between 1900 and 1950*: Brigham Bastian et al., "Mortality Trends in the United States, 1900–2018," National Center for Health Statistics, 2020, https://www.cdc.gov/nchs/data-visualization/mortality-trends/index.htm.

34 *the average American life spanned sixty-eight years*: Robert H. Shmerling, "Why Life Expectancy in the US Is Falling," *Harvard Health Publishing*, October 20,

2022, https://www.health.harvard.edu/blog/why-life-expectancy-in-the-us-is-falling-202210202835.

35 *By the year 2000, the leading causes of death*: Bastian et al., "Mortality Trends."

35 *the life expectancy in the United States*: Elizabeth Arias, "United States Life Tables, 2000," *National Vital Statistics Reports* 19, no. 3 (December 2002): 1–38.

36 *"We have a wonderful sick-care system"*: "Transcript: Explaining America with Asaf Bitton and Michelle A. Williams," *Washington Post Live, Washington Post*, April 10, 2023, https://www.washingtonpost.com/washington-post-live/2023/04/10/transcript-explaining-america-with-asaf-bitton-michelle-williams/.

36 *One multilevel analysis done*: Amy J. Schulz et al., "Associations Between Socioeconomic Status and Allostatic Load: Effects of Neighborhood Poverty and Tests of Mediating Pathways," *American Journal of Public Health* 102, no. 9 (September 2012): 1706–14, https://doi.org/10.2105/AJPH.2011.300412.

37 *Other studies have revealed similar findings*: Andrew Steptoe et al., "Disruption of Multisystem Responses to Stress in Type 2 Diabetes: Investigating the Dynamics of Allostatic Load," *Proceedings of the National Academy of Sciences* 111, no. 44 (October 20, 2014): 15693–98, https://doi.org/10.1073/pnas.1410401111.

37 *Black teen mothers*: Arline T. Geronimus, "The Weathering Hypothesis and the Health of African-American Women and Infants: Evidence and Speculations," *Ethnicity and Disease* 2, no. 3 (Summer 1992): 207–21.

37 *celebrated for providing a framework*: Alisha Haridasani Gupta, "How 'Weathering' Contributes to Racial Health Disparities," *New York Times*, April 12, 2023, https://www.nytimes.com/2023/04/12/well/live/weathering-health-racism-discrimination.html.

37 *In 2023, Geronimus published* Weathering: Arline T. Geronimus, *Weathering: The Extraordinary Stress of Ordinary Life in an Unjust Society* (New York: Hachette, 2023).

Chapter 3: Accept Your Current Situation

49 *Anguished, he shouted out*: Steven Hayes, "Psychological Flexibility: How Love Turns Pain into Purpose," TEDxUniversityofNevada, February 22, 2016, https://www.youtube.com/watch?v=o79_gmO5ppg.

49 *They found that ACT*: Andrew T. Gloster et al., "The Empirical Status of Acceptance and Commitment Therapy: A Review of Meta-Analyses," *Journal of Contextual Behavioral Science* 21 (July 2021): 223–26, https://doi.org/10.1016/j.jcbs.2020.09.009.

49 *And this study is just part*: Xiaohuan Jin et al., "Acceptance and Commitment Therapy for Psychological and Behavioural Changes Among Parents of Children with Chronic Health Conditions: A Systematic Review," *Journal of Advanced Nursing* 77, no. 7 (July 2021): 3020–33, https://doi.org/10.1111/jan.14798.

49 *to heathcare workers reporting distress*: Arianna Prudenzi et al., "Group-Based Acceptance and Commitment Therapy Interventions for Improving General Distress and Work-Related Distress in Healthcare Professionals: A Systematic

Notes

Review and Meta-Analysis," *Journal of Affective Disorders* 295 (December 1, 2021): 192–202, https://doi.org/10.1016/j.jad.2021.07.084.

52 *She then asks the audience to look at the room*: Lucy Hone, "Three Secrets of Resilient People," TEDxChristchurch, August 2019, https://www.ted.com/talks/lucy_hone_3_secrets_of_resilient_people.

54 *She underlined again*: "Latest Research on the Study of Resilience and One Couple's Personal Story," *CBS Mornings*, August 11, 2021, https://www.youtube.com/watch?v=t1BCp_VRjh4.

Chapter 4: Embrace Flexible Thinking

66 *In 1990, the World Health Organization*: Vyjeyanthi S. Periyakoil and Charles F. von Gunten, "Palliative Care Is Proven," *Journal of Palliative Medicine* 26, no. 1 (December 30, 2022): 2–4, https://doi.org/10.1089/jpm.2022.0568.

66 *Not until 2006*: "ABMS Boards to Offer Certification in Hospice and Palliative Care Medicine," Center to Advance Palliative Care, January 16, 2007, https://www.capc.org/about/press-media/press-releases/2007-1-16/abms-boards-offer-certification-hospice-and-palliative-care-medicine/.

67 *The analysis of multiple systematic reviews*: Jiaxin Cui et al., "Meta-Analysis of Effects of Early Palliative Care on Health-Related Outcomes Among Advanced Cancer Patients," *Nursing Research* 72, no. 6 (2023), https://doi.org/10.1097/NNR.0000000000000687.

73 *Now that we know how we're feeling*: Steven Hayes, "The Most Important Skill Set in Mental Health," Steven C. Hayes, PhD, https://stevenchayes.com/the-most-important-skill-set-in-mental-health-2/.

74 *Cohen, who called the book a "reluctant memoir,"* : Richard M. Cohen, *Blindsided: Lifting a Life Above Illness* (New York: Harper Perennial, 2005).

78 *Beecher found that in fifteen trials*: Gunver S. Kienle and Helmut Kiene, "The Powerful Placebo Effect: Fact or Fiction?," *Journal of Clinical Epidemiology* 50, no. 12 (December 1997): 1311–18, https://doi.org/10.1016/S0895-4356(97)00203-5.

78 *Incredibly, the two groups*: J. Bruce Moseley et al., "A Controlled Trial of Arthroscopic Surgery for Osteoarthritis of the Knee," *New England Journal of Medicine* 347, no. 2 (July 11, 2002): 81–88, https://www.doi.org/10.1056/NEJMoa013259.

80 *Crum and Langer published their findings*: Alia J. Crum and Ellen J. Langer, "Mind-Set Matters: Exercise and the Placebo Effect," *Psychological Science* 18, no. 2 (February 2007): 165–71, https://doi.org/10.1111/j.1467-9280.2007.01867.x.

81 *The difference in ghrelin production and levels was significant*: Alia J. Crum and William R. Corbin, "Mind over Milkshakes: Mindsets, Not Just Nutrients, Determine Ghrelin Response," *Health Psychology* 30, no. 4 (2001): 424–29, https://psycnet.apa.org/doi/10.1037/a0023467.

83 *When patients anticipate adverse effects*: Patricia Rosenberger et al., "Psychosocial Factors and Surgical Outcomes: An Evidence-Based Literature Review," *Journal*

Notes

of the American Academy of Orthopaedic Surgeons 14, no. 7 (July 2006): 397–405, https://www.doi.org/10.5435/00124635-200607000-00002.

83 *Or, when a brand-name drug*: Kate Faasse and Leslie R. Martin, "The Power of Labeling in Nocebo Effects," *International Review of Neurobiology* 139 (2018): 379–406, https://doi.org/10.1016/bs.irn.2018.07.016.

84 *"stress makes you sick"*: Kelly McGonigal, "How to Make Stress Your Friend," TEDGlobal 2013, June 2013, https://www.ted.com/talks/kelly_mcgonigal_how_to_make_stress_your_friend?language=en.

84 *Participants who reported*: Abiola Keller et al., "Does the Perception That Stress Affects Health Matter? The Association with Health and Mortality," *Health Psychology* 31, no. 5 (2012): 677–84, https://doi.org/10.1037/a0026743.

Chapter 5: Get Fit

90 *Unsurprisingly, many of these patients*: Julie Redfern et al., "Historical Context of Cardiac Rehabilitation: Learning from the Past to Move to the Future," *Frontiers in Cardiovascular Medicine* 9 (2022), https://doi.org/10.3389/fcvm.2022.842567.

91 *His insistence that cardiac patients*: "Dr. Bernard Lown," Lown Institute, November 19, 2021, https://lowninstitute.org/about/dr-bernard-lown/.

91 *Lown conducted what is now immortalized*: Leslie S. Leighton, "The Story of the 'Cardiac Chair' and the Resistance to Its Use in Patients with Acute Myocardial Infarction, 1950 to 1961," *American Journal of Cardiology* 120, no. 9 (November 2017): 1674–80, https://doi.org/10.1016/j.amjcard.2017.07.070.

91 *in an interview recorded in 2010*: Judith Garber, "Lessons from Lown: How the Levine Chair Changed Heart Attack Treatment Forever," Lown Institute, April 6, 2021, https://lowninstitute.org/lessons-from-lown-how-the-levine-chair-changed-heart-attack-treatment-forever/.

92 *He was not only focused on "protecting" the heart after a trauma*: Ibid.

92 *a fan of bicycling*: Siang Yong Tan and Erika Kwock, "Paul Dudley White (1886–1973): Pioneer in Modern Cardiology," *Singapore Medical Journal* 57, no. 4 (2015): 215–16, https://www.doi.org/10.11622/smedj.2016075.

92 *The work of researchers such as Dr. Herman Hellerstein*: Herman K. Hellerstein, "Exercise Therapy in Coronary Disease," *Bulletin of the New York Academy of Medicine* 44, no. 8 (August 1968): 1028–47, https://pmc.ncbi.nlm.nih.gov/articles/PMC1750285/pdf/bullnyacadmed00245-0142.pdf.

93 *During these sessions, researchers noticed*: Julie Redfern et al., "Historical Context of Cardiac Rehabilitation: Learning from the Past to Move to the Future," *Frontiers in Cardiovascular Medicine* 9 (2022), https://doi.org/10.3389/fcvm.2022.842567.

93 *It also helps regulate immune cells*: Ken Kingery, "Exercising Muscle Combats Chronic Inflammation on Its Own," Duke Pratt School of Engineering, January 22, 2021, https://pratt.duke.edu/news/exercise-muscle-inflammation.

93 *The American Heart Association recommends*: "American Heart Association Recommendations for Physical Activity in Adults and Kids," American Heart

Notes

Association, https://www.heart.org/en/healthy-living/fitness/fitness-basics/aha-recs-for-physical-activity-in-adults.

94 *A study published*: Yanghui Liu et al., "Associations of Resistance Exercise with Cardiovascular Disease Morbidity and Mortality," *Medicine & Science in Sports & Exercise* 51, no. 3 (March 2019): 499–508, https://www.doi.org/10.1249/MSS.0000000000001822.

94 *In effect, myokines*: Kelly McGonigal, *The Joy of Movement: How Exercise Helps Us Find Happiness, Hope, Connection, and Courage* (New York: Avery, 2019).

101 *Johns Hopkins researchers measured*: Chiadi D. Ndumele et al., "Obesity, Subclinical Myocardial Injury, and Incident Heart Failure," *JACC: Heart Failure* 2, no. 6 (2014): 715, https://doi.org/10.1016/j.jchf.2014.05.017.

106 *The doctors in the on-call group*: Jose Morales et al., "Stress and Autonomic Response to Sleep Deprivation in Medical Residents: A Comparative Cross-Sectional Study," *PLoS One* 14, no. 4 (April 4, 2019), https://doi.org/10.1371/journal.pone.0214858.

107 *Use a blue-light filter*: Lisa Howard, "Try These 13 Tips to Help You Sleep Better," UC Davis Health, July 10, 2023, https://health.ucdavis.edu/news/headlines/try-these-13-tips-to-help-you-sleep-better/2023/07.

108 *A study on habit formation*: Phillippa Lally et al., "Experiences of Habit Formation: A Qualitative Study," *Psychology, Health & Medicine* 16, no. 4 (2011): 48–89, https://doi.org/10.1080/13548506.2011.555774.

111 *A statement entitled*: Glenn N. Levine et al., "Psychological Health, Well-Being, and the Mind-Heart-Body Connection: A Scientific Statement from the American Heart Association," *Circulation* 143, no. 10 (January 25, 2021), https://doi.org/10.1161/CIR.0000000000000947.

114 *around eight hundred thousand*: "Heart Disease Facts," Centers for Disease Control, October 24, 2024, https://www.cdc.gov/heart-disease/data-research/facts-stats/index.html.

114 *Studies have found*: Jessica T. Servey and Mark Stephens, "Cardiac Rehabilitation: Improving Function and Reducing Risk," *American Family Physician* 94, no. 1 (2016): 37–43.

114 *The mental benefits*: "How Cardiac Rehabilitation Can Help Heal Your Heart," Centers for Disease Control, May 24, 2024, https://www.cdc.gov/heart-disease/about/cardiac-rehabilitation-treatment.html.

114 *Cardiac rehabilitation programs*: Servey and Stephens, "Cardiac Rehabilitation," 37–43.

Chapter 6: Face Your Fear

117 *A headline from the American Heart Association*: "Fear of Another Heart Attack May Be a Major Source of Ongoing Stress for Survivors," American Heart Association, November 11, 2024, https://newsroom.heart.org/news/fear-of-another-heart-attack-may-be-a-major-source-of-ongoing-stress-for-survivors?preview=c947&preview_mode=True.

Notes

118 *controlling for depression and anxiety*: Sarah Zvonar et al., "Fear of Recurrence in Acute Myocardial Infarction Survivors," *Circulation* 150, no. 1 (November 11, 2024), https://doi.org/10.1161/circ.150.suppl_1.4144762.

118 *Sixty volunteers prone to anxiety*: Michael W. Otto et al., "Exercise for Mood and Anxiety Disorders," *Primary Care Companion to The Journal of Clinical Psychiatry* 9, no. 4 (2007): 287–94, https://www.doi.org/10.4088/pcc.v09n0406.

118 *"People learn to associate"*: Kirsten Weir, "The Exercise Effect," *Monitor on Psychology* 42, no. 11 (2011), https://www.apa.org/monitor/2011/12/exercise.

120 *Are we being chased*: "Fear," Paul Ekman Group, August 15, 2024, https://www.paulekman.com/universal-emotions/what-is-fear/.

122 *I definitely feel*: "Kelly McGonigal: Can We Reframe the Way We Think About Stress?," NPR, August 2, 2019, https://www.npr.org/transcripts/747384008?t=1639652981049&t=1643646142486.

123 *Walter Cannon*: Esther M. Sternberg, "Walter B. Cannon and 'Voodoo' Death: A Perspective from 60 Years On," *American Journal of Public Health* 92, no. 10 (October 2002): 1564–66, https://www.doi.org/ https://doi.org/10.2105/ajph.92.10.1564.

123 *Samuels and his team*: Martin A. Samuels, "The Brain-Heart Connection," *Circulation* 166, no. 1 (July 3, 2007), https://doi.org/10.1161/CIRCULATIONAHA.106.678995.

123 *Right there on the golf course*: "Scared to Death . . . Literally," NPR, October 26, 2012, https://www.npr.org/2012/10/26/163712863/scared-to-death-literally.

127 *The good news*: Rich Diviney, "The Psychology of Fear; Understand the Triggers That Cause It, Why We Ignore It, and How to Overcome It," *Attributes*, July 25, 2022, https://theattributes.com/blog/the-psychology-of-fear.

133 *American psychologist David Barlow*: Martin M. Antony et al., "Current Perspectives on Panic and Panic Disorder," *Current Directions in Psychological Science* 1, no. 3 (June 1992): 79–82, https://doi.org/10.1111/1467-8721.ep10768720.

Chapter 7: Build Connections

142 *This is the philosophy*: Angela M. Hicks and Carolyn Korbel, "Attachment Theory," in *Encyclopedia of Behavioral Medicine*, ed. M. D. Gellman and J. R. Turner (New York: Springer, 2013), 149–55.

142 *Perhaps you've heard about*: Paul Main, "Bowlby's Attachment Theory," Structural Learning, June 30, 2023, https://www.structural-learning.com/post/bowlbys-attachment-theory.

142 *These children often did not*: Ibid.

147 *In a coauthored review*: John T. Cacioppo et al., "Social Isolation," *Annals of the New York Academy of Sciences* 1231, no. 1 (June 8, 2011): 17–22, https://doi.org/10.1111/j.1749-6632.2011.06028.x.

149 *This reduced flexibility*: Bruno B. Lima et al., "Association of Transient Endothelial Dysfunction Induced by Mental Stress with Major Adverse Cardiovascular Events in Men and Women with Coronary Artery Disease,"

Notes

JAMA Cardiology 4, no. 10 (2019): 988–96, https://jamanetwork.com/journals/jamacardiology/fullarticle/2749539.

152 *Data from the National Poll on Healthy Aging*: Kevin Gavin, "1 in 3 Older Adults Still Experience Loneliness and Isolation," Michigan Medicine, December 9, 2024, https://www.michiganmedicine.org/health-lab/1-3-older-adults-still-experience-loneliness-and-isolation.

152 *Alarmingly, a report*: Ibid.

153 *According to a March 2024 Allconnect report*: Camryn Smith, "The Average Adult Spends over Seven Hours Online—Here's How You Can Manage Your Screen Time," Allconnect, February 23, 2024, https://www.allconnect.com/blog/screen-time-stats.

153 *In a February 2023 study*: Christine Anderl et al., "Directly Measured Smartphone Screen Time Predicts Well-Being and Feelings of Social Connectedness," *Journal of Social and Personal Relationships* 41, no. 5 (2023): 1073–90, https://doi.org/10.1177/02654075231158300.

156 *The phrase* find, remind, and bind: Sara B. Algoe, "Find, Remind, and Bind: The Functions of Gratitude in Everyday Relationships," *Social and Personality Psychology Compass* 6, no. 6 (May 2012): 455–69, https://doi.org/10.1111/j.1751-9004.2012.00439.x.

159 *A study done in the middle of the COVID pandemic*: Kaveri Subrahmanyam et al., "The Relation Between Face-to-Face and Digital Interactions and Self-Esteem: A Daily Diary Study," *Human Behavior and Emerging Technology* 2, no. 2 (March 2020): 116–27, https://doi.org/10.1002/hbe2.187.

Chapter 8: Seek Out Love

172 *Even more interesting*: Emelia Watts et al., "The Role of Compassionate Care in Medicine: Toward Improving Patients' Quality of Care and Satisfaction," *Journal of Surgical Research* 289 (September 2023): 1–7, https://doi.org/10.1016/j.jss.2023.03.024.

172 *For example, one study found*: Jorge Moll et al., "Human Fronto-Mesolimbic Networks Guide Decisions About Charitable Donation," *PNAS* 103, no. 42 (October 2006): 15623–28, https://doi.org/10.1073/pnas.0604475103.

173 *Another study showed*: "A General Benevolence Dimension That Links Neural, Psychological, Economic, and Life-Span Data on Altruistic Tendencies": Correction to Hubbard et al. (2016), *Journal of Experimental Psychology: General* 145, no. 10 (October 2016): 1358, https://doi.org/10.1037/xge0000235.

173 *People who had happy marriages*: Robert J. Waldinger and Marc S. Schulz, "What's Love Got to Do with It?: Social Functioning, Perceived Health, and Daily Happiness in Married Octogenarians," *Psychology and Aging* 25, no. 2 (2010): 422–31, https://doi.org/10.1037/a0019087.

177 *A study conducted*: J. Robin Moon et al., "Short- and Long-Term Associations Between Widowhood and Mortality in the United States: Longitudinal

Notes

Analyses," *Journal of Public Health* 36, no. 3 (September 2014): 382–89, https://doi.org/10.1093/pubmed/fdt101.

177 *Even more astounding*: Iain M. Carey et al., "Increased Risk of Acute Cardiovascular Events After Partner Bereavement: A Matched Cohort Study," *JAMA Internal Medicine* 174, no. 4 (April 2014): 598–605, doi:10.1001/jamainternmed.2013.14558.

177 *This added to a study*: Elizabeth Mostofsky et al., "Risk of Acute Myocardial Infarction After the Death of a Significant Person in One's Life: The Determinants of Myocardial Infarction Onset Study," *Circulation* 125, no. 3 (January 2012), https://doi.org/10.1161/CIRCULATIONAHA.111.061770.

179 *More than 90 percent*: "Takotsubo Cardiomyopathy—Symptoms, Causes, Treatment," National Organization for Rare Disorders, accessed April 4, 2025, https://rarediseases.org/rare-diseases/takotsubo-cardiomyopathy/.

180 *In a 2009 study*: Matthew J. Hertenstein et al., "The Communication of Emotion via Touch," *Emotion* 9, no. 4 (2009): 566–73, https://doi.org/10.1037/a0016108.

180 *A 2021 study*: Aljoscha Dreisoerner et al., "Self-Soothing Touch and Being Hugged Reduce Cortisol Responses to Stress: A Randomized Controlled Trial on Stress, Physical Touch, and Social Identity," *Comprehensive Psychoneuroendocrinology* 8 (November 2021), https://doi.org/10.1016/j.cpnec.2021.100091.

181 *Holding hands with a loved one*: "Hand-Holding 'Supportive Touch' Leads to Less Pain," PainWeek, July 2, 2019, https://www.painweek.org/media/news/hand-holding-supportive-touch-leads-less-pain.

182 *self-compassion was positively*: F. M. Sirois, R. Kitner, and J. K. Hirsch, "Self-Compassion, Affect, and Health-Promoting Behaviors," *Health Psychology* 34, no. 6 (2015): 661–69, https://doi.org/10.1037/hea0000158.

183 *Or another published in 2020*: Amanda Davey, et al., "Psychological Flexibility, Self-Compassion and Daily Functioning in Chronic Pain," *Journal of Contextual Behavioral Science* 17 (July 2020): 79–85.

183 *Of particular interest*: Rebecca C. Thurston et al., "Self-Compassion and Subclinical Cardiovascular Disease Among Midlife Women," *Health Psychology* 40, no. 11 (2021): 747–53, https://psycnet.apa.org/doi/10.1037/hea0001137.

183 *These statements range*: Kristin Neff, "Development and Validation of a Scale to Measure Self-Compassion," *Self and Identity* 2 (2003): 223–50, https://self-compassion.org/wp-content/uploads/2021/03/SCS-information.pdf.

183 *These participants with more self-compassion*: Thurston et al., "Self-Compassion," 747–53.

183 *The World Health Organization defines self-care*: "Self-Care for Health and Well-Being," World Health Organization, April 26, 2024, https://www.who.int/news-room/fact-sheets/detail/self-care-health-interventions.

184 *A Healthy Cities initiative*: Hugh Barton et al., "Health Urban Planning in European Cities," *Health Promotion International* 24 (November 2009): i91–i199, https://www. https://doi.org/10.1093/heapro/dap059.

Notes

184 *In a 2017 study*: Barbara Riegel et al., "Self-Care for the Prevention and Management of Cardiovascular Disease and Stroke: A Scientific Statement for Healthcare Professionals from the American Heart Association," *Journal of the American Heart Association* 6, no. 9 (August 2017), https://doi.org/10.1161/JAHA.117.006997.

Chapter 9: Finding Hope and Having Faith

193 *Research into hope's relationship*: Charles R. Snyder et al., "Hope for Rehabilitation and Vice Versa," *Rehabilitation Psychology* 51, no. 2 (2006): 89–112, https://psycnet.apa.org/doi/10.1037/0090-5550.51.2.89.

194 *A few key findings*: Katelyn N. G. Long et al., "The Role of Hope in Subsequent Health and Well-Being for Older Adults: An Outcome-Wise Longitudinal Approach," *Global Epidemiology* 2 (November 2020), https://doi.org/10.1016/j.gloepi.2020.100018.

195 *Another study published*: Corine Nierop-van Baalen et al., "Associated Factors of Hope in Cancer Patients during Treatment: A Systematic Literature Review," *Journal of Advanced Nursing* 76, no. 7 (July 2020): 1520–1537, https://doi.org/10.1111/jan.14344.

196 *"There have been countless moments"*: Brenda Gazzar, "City of Hope's Alexandra Levine Leads the Way in Medical Research, Compassionate Care," *Los Angeles Daily News*, August 28, 2017, https://www.dailynews.com/2012/12/11/city-of-hopes-alexandra-levine-leads-the-way-in-medical-research-compassionate-care/.

199 *Attendance also reduced*: Raphael Bonelli et al., "Religious and Spiritual Factors in Depression: Review and Integration of the Research," *Depression Research and Treatment* 2012, no. 1 (2012), https://doi.org/10.1155/2012/962860.

200 *Research has also demonstrated*: Kenneth I. Pargament et al., "Religious Coping Methods as Predictors of Psychological, Physical and Spiritual Outcomes Among Medically Ill Elderly Patients: A Two-year Longitudinal Study," *Journal of Health Psychology* 9, no. 6 (November 2004): 713–30, https://doi.org/10.1177/1359105304045366.

200 *A study published*: Tyler J. VanderWeele et al., "Attendance at Religious Services, Prayer, Religious Coping, and Religious/Spiritual Identity as Predictors of All-Cause Mortality in the Black Women's Health Study," *American Journal of Epidemiology* 185, no. 7 (April 2017), https://doi.org/10.1093/aje/kww179.

201 *In one study*: Nathan L. Henry and Nathan Gilley, "Spiritual Assessment," StatPearls (Treasure Island, FL: StatPearls Publishing), January 2024.

201 *The number increased*: Ibid.

201 *despite these desires*: Ibid.

202 *Furthermore, the data reveals*: Harold G. Koenig, "Religion, Spirituality, and Health: The Research and Clinical Implications," *ISRN Psychiatry* 2012, no. 1 (December 2012), https://doi.org/10.5402/2012/278730.

Notes

202 *That in patient-centered care*: Tracy A. Balboni et al., "Spirituality in Serious Illness and Health," *JAMA* 328, no. 2 (2022): 184–97, https://www.doi.org/10.1001/jama.2022.11086.

202 *As Koh put it*: "Spirituality Linked with Better Health Outcomes, Patient Care," Harvard T. H. Chan School of Public Health, July 12, 2022, https://hsph.harvard.edu/news/spirituality-better-health-outcomes-patient-care/.

Chapter 10: Pursue Your Purpose

221 *A more recent test*: Gitima Sharma et al., "Sense of Purpose Scale: Development and Initial Validation," *Applied Developmental Science* 22, no. 3 (2018): 188–99, https://doi.org/10.1080/10888691.2016.1262262.

223 *Adults with a greater sense of purpose*: Glenn N. Levine et al., "Psychological Health, Well-Being, and the Mind-Heart-Body Connection: A Scientific Statement from the American Heart Association," *Circulation* 143, no. 10 (January 2021), https://doi.org/10.1161/CIR.0000000000000947.

223 *Findings showed*: Randy Cohen et al., "Purpose in Life and Its Relationship to All-Cause Mortality and Cardiovascular Events: A Meta-Analysis," *Psychosomatic Medicine* 78, no. 2 (February/March 2016): 122–33, https://www.doi.org/10.1097/PSY.0000000000000274.

224 *As noted in a 2018 study*: Patrick L. Hill et al., "Sense of Purpose Moderates the Associations Between Daily Stressors and Daily Well-Being," *Annals of Behavioral Medicine* 52, no. 8 (August 2018): 724–29, https://doi.org/10.1093/abm/kax039.

224 *Though the results are inconclusive*: Mariangela Boccardi and Virginia Boccardi, "Psychological Wellbeing and Healthy Aging: Focus on Telomeres," *Geriatrics* (Basel) 4, no. 1 (February 2019), https://doi.org/10.3390/geriatrics4010025.

227 *The World Health Organization describes*: "Burn-Out an 'Occupational Phenomenon': International Classification of Diseases," World Health Organization, May 28, 2019, https://www.who.int/news/item/28-05-2019-burn-out-an-occupational-phenomenon-international-classification-of-diseases.

228 *Researchers affiliated*: Tait D. Shanafelt et al., "Changes in Burnout and Satisfaction with Work-Life Integration in Physicians During the First 2 Years of the COVID-19 Pandemic," *Mayo Clinic Proceedings* 97, no. 12 (December 2022): 2248–58, https://doi.org/10.1016/j.mayocp.2022.09.002.

229 *According to Definitive Healthcare*: "Addressing the Healthcare Staffing Shortage," Definitive Healthcare, https://www.definitivehc.com/resources/research/healthcare-staffing-shortage.

229 *physician demand will*: GlobalData Plc. The Complexities of Physician Supply and Demand: Projections From 2021 to 2036. Washington, DC: AAMC; 2024.

229 *projected that by this year*: Rahulkumar Singh et al., "Provider Burnout." StatPearls (Treasure Island, FL: StatPearls Publishing), 2023.

Notes

229 *The problem is so dire*: "Addressing Health Worker Burnout: The U.S. Surgeon General's Advisory on Building a Thriving Health Workforce," Office of the US Surgeon General, US Department of Health and Human Services, 2022, https://www.hhs.gov/sites/default/files/health-worker-wellbeing-advisory.pdf.

230 *In a 2022 survey*: Young Kyun Chang et al., "Profit or Purpose: What Increases Medical Doctors' Job Satisfaction?," *Healthcare* (Basel) 10, no. 4 (March 2022), https://doi.org/10.3390/healthcare10040641.

231 *Sakran told him*: Simar Bajaj, "He Was Shot in the Throat. Now He Saves Gun Victims as a Trauma Surgeon in Baltimore," *Guardian*, June 20, 2024, https://www.theguardian.com/us-news/ng-interactive/2024/jun/20/gun-wound-trauma-surgeon-doctor-joseph-sakran.

231 *When Sakran saw*: Ibid.

232 *those who participated in these workshops*: Carol R. Horowitz et al., "What Do Doctors Find Meaningful About Their Work?," *Annals of Internal Medicine* 138, no. 9 (May 2003): 772–75, https://doi.org/10.7326/0003-4819-138-9-200305060-00028.

232 *One of its chief recommendations*: "Addressing Health Worker Burnout," Office of the US Surgeon General.

232 *The AMA even established*: "Joy in Medicine Health System Recognition Program—2025 Program Guidelines," American Medical Association, 2024, https://www.ama-assn.org/system/files/joy-in-medicine-guidelines.pdf.

232 *establish leadership roles*: Ibid.

233 *When asked about*: Michael S. Sinha, "Dr. Sinha: The Moment I Knew Medicine Was My Calling," American Medical Association, May 8, 2017, https://www.ama-assn.org/practice-management/physician-health/dr-sinha-moment-i-knew-medicine-was-my-calling.

233 *"Thus, I chose the alternate"*: Fatima Cody Stanford, "Dr. Stanford: The Moment I Knew Medicine Was My Calling," American Medical Association, May 29, 2017, https://www.ama-assn.org/practice-management/physician-health/dr-stanford-moment-i-knew-medicine-was-my-calling.

Index

ABC News, 74, 219
acceptance, 41–61
   after medical diagnosis, 41–45, 48–51
   in grief and loss, 51–61. *see also* grief
   palliative care and, 66
   radical acceptance, 171–72
   resiliency stories of, 2, 45–48, 5 5–56
acceptance and commitment therapy (ACT), 45, 49–50
acute stress, 20–21, 25–26, 33, 35
adaptive calibration, 8–9
adrenaline, 20, 24, 56–57, 123, 124, 149, 179
adrenocorticotropic hormone, 19–20
Adult Hope Scale (AHS), 193–94
adversity, in building resilience, 8–11, 27, 136–37
aerobic exercise, 30, 32, 93–94
agency, in theory of hope, 193
Aguirre, Aitor, 181–82
Ahmed, Robert, 230–31
alcohol use, 90, 107, 223, 225
Allconnect, on screen time (2024), 153
allostatic load, 36–37
ambiguous loss, 60–61
American Board of Medical Specialties, 66
American College of Physicians, 231–32

American Heart Association. *see also* cardiovascular disease
   co-founder of, 92
   on CVD as leading cause of death, 17
   on exercise guidelines, 30, 93. *see also* exercise and fitness
   Go Red for Women, 163
   on heart attack recurrence fear, 117–18
   on heart attack risk after loved one's death, 177
   on high blood pressure, 97. *see also* hypertension
   on mental health and CVD, 18–19, 111
   on sleep as critical lifestyle factor, 106
American Institute for Cognitive Therapy (New York), 134
American Journal of Epidemiology, 200
American Medical Association (AMA), 172, 228, 232–33
amygdala, 19–20, 25, 29, 120, 124, 149
The Annals of Behavioral Medicine, 224
Annals of the New York Academy of Sciences, 147
Anne (resiliency story), 1–3, 5–6, 217
anxiety
   ambiguous loss and, 60
   chronic stress and, 25
   exercise role in avoiding panic, 117–18
   fear vs., 133–34

Index

anxiety (*cont.*)
  loneliness effect on, 147
  religious/spiritual practices and, 199, 202
  sleep deprivation and, 105
  therapies for, 49, 118–19, 134–36
Applied Developmental Science (journal), 221–22
arrhythmia (irregular heartbeat), 57
Association of American Medical Colleges, 229
atherosclerosis (plaque buildup), 32, 33, 44, 131, 149
attachment theory, 142, 158–59, 219–20
autonomic nervous system, 19, 156

Balboni, Tracy, 202
Barlow, David, 133–36
Beck, Aaron, 193
Beck Hopelessness Scale, 193
Beecher, Henry K., 78
Before and After Loss (Shulman), 179
Bitton, Asaf, 36
Black patients, healthcare inequities and, 16
Black Women's Health Study, 16
Blindsided: Lifting a Life Above Illness (Cohen), 74, 76
blockages, xiii, 18, 32, 130, 203–4
blood clotting, chronic stress and, 33
blood pressure
  adrenaline effect on, 149
  lifestyle changes and, 33, 38–40
  loneliness effect on, 147, 149
  monitoring of, 130–31, 184
  oxytocin in lowering, 180, 181
  preeclampsia patient, 136
  protective dip during sleep, 106–7
  readings of, 96–97
blood vessels, 33, 94, 97, 149, 179, 181
body mass index (BMI), 99–101
Bonanno, George, 11–12, 26–27, 29
Bowlby, John, 142, 158–59
Brach, Tara, 171–72

brain
  cardiac health and, 123
  compassion effects on, 172–73
  excitement response and, 124
  exercise benefits for, 93
  in fight, flight, or freeze response, 19–20, 120
  grief effects on, 177–79
  loneliness effects on, 149, 151
  myokines and mood, 94–95
  nutrition and, 102
  sleep essential to, 104–5
  stress effects on, 22–30
breathing exercises, 45, 107, 185
Brigham and Women's Hospital (Boston), 123, 143, 179, 233
broken heart syndrome, xiii, 179–80
Brown University School of Medicine, 200
building connections, 139–65. *see also* loneliness and social isolation
  finding sense of purpose, 226–27
  fostering warm connections, 155–60, 164–65
  group activities in, 163
  loneliness effects on mind and body, 146–55
  in medical settings, 143–46, 232
  resiliency story, 139–41
  secure and healthy attachment in, 141–43, 158–59
  self-care and, 186
  through grief, 179
  value of support network in healing, 4, 170–71
burnout, 227–30, 232

Cacioppo, John, 146–48
caffeine, 105, 107
calcium score, 124–25
Calhoun, Lawrence, 10–11, 12
cancer, 50–51, 100–102, 191–92, 195–96
Cannon, Walter, 123
carbohydrates, 100, 102

Index

cardiac catheterization, 32, 88–89
cardiac electrophysiology, xiv, 213
cardiac rehabilitation, 92–93, 114–15, 184
cardiac stress tests, 31–32
cardiac tone, acute stress and, 33
cardiophobia, 122
cardiovascular disease (CVD)
    accepting difficult diagnosis, 41–45
    ambiguous loss and, 60
    calcium score and, 124–25
    chronic stress and, 33–34
    grief and, 177
    lifestyle choices and, 17, 30–31, 32–33, 87. *see also* lifestyle choices
    loneliness and risk of, 148–49, 151
    mental health and, 18–19, 111
    misdiagnosis of, 41–42
    prevalence and mortality of, xiii, 17
    resiliency stories, 1–3, 5–6, 31–33, 124–26, 198, 203–4
    self-compassion and risk factors for, 183
    sense of purpose and, 223–24
    sleep deprivation and, 105–7
    weight and heart-muscle injury, 101
cardioverter, 43, 91
carotid intima-media thickness (IMT), 183
Cath Lab. *see* cardiac catheterization
Cathy (resiliency story), 124–26
CBS News, 53, 88, 219, 225, 233
CBT. *see* cognitive behavioral therapy
Center for the Vulnerable Child (University of Southern California), 144–45
Centers for Disease Control and Prevention (CDC), 114
chair experiment, heart attack care and, 91–92
Chan School of Public Health (Harvard University), 36
Charles (resiliency story), 139–41, 146
Charney, Dennis, 12–15, 228–29
chest pain, 18, 32, 88

children
    attachment theory and, 142, 158–59
    bond with parents, 188–89
    resilience development in, 8–10, 15
    sense of purpose in, 219–20
cholesterol levels, 33, 42, 100
Chris (resiliency story), 130–32
chronic disease
    increase in, 34–38
    inflammation and, 93, 100
    obesity as, 109–10
    sleep deprivation and, 105, 107
chronic pain, 49, 183, 195
chronic stress
    brain function and, 24–25
    health risks of, 20–22, 33–35
    loneliness as, 148–49, 151
    obesity and, 110
    sense of purpose and, 224
    sleep deprivation and, 105
    societal inequities and, 36–38
circadian rhythm, 19, 148
Circulation (journal), 30, 223, 225
City of Hope (Los Angeles), 195–97
Claudia (resiliency story), 71–72
cognitive behavioral therapy (CBT), 28, 49, 134–36, 179, 193
cognitive flexibility, 13
cognitive narrowing, 120
cognitive reframing, 137–38
cognitive restructuring, 136
Cohen, Richard, 73–77
"compare and despair," 161
compassion, 172–73, 180
conserved transcriptional response to adversity (CTRA), 148
coping mechanisms, 8, 13, 39–40, 134, 136, 199, 200
coronary artery disease, 22, 32, 101, 203
corticotropin-releasing hormone (CRH), 19, 148
cortisol, 16, 20, 24, 93, 105–6, 110, 148, 158, 181, 224

Index

courage, 126–27
COVID pandemic
  burnout in healthcare profession and, 227–29
  increase in loneliness increase since, 152
  resilience center as response to, 14–15
  screen time increase since, 153
  short- and long-term effects of, 22
Croix, Gwendolyn La, 225
Crum, Alia, on placebo effect, 79–82
CVD. *see* cardiovascular disease

Dalai Lama, 172
DASH diet (Dietary Approaches to Stop Hypertension), 103
Dean Charney Award for Resilience, 14
death, facing fear of, 128–29. *see also* mortality
decision-making, 25, 29, 105
Definitive Healthcare, 229
Department of Psychiatry and Behavioral Sciences (UC Davis), 107–8
DePierro, Jonathan, 137–38, 164–65
depression
  after heart attack, 118
  ambiguous loss and, 60
  cardiac rehabilitation and, 114
  chronic stress and, 25
  face-to-face contact in mitigating, 159
  religious/spiritual practices and, 199–200, 202
  sleep deprivation and, 105
  therapies for, 49
  weight-related, 101, 102
Depression Research and Treatment (journal), 199–200
diabetes, 22, 37, 89, 100, 151
diastolic blood pressure, 97, 184
diet. *see* nutrition and diet
digestive system function, 20, 102, 103, 148
Diviney, Rich, 127
divorce, 11, 51, 60
dizziness, 42, 56

doctors and healthcare providers. *see also* Narula, Tara
  building connections with patients and colleagues, 143–46, 232
  compassionate care and, 172
  COVID and burnout in, 227–29
  discussing patients' faith and beliefs, 200–204
  doctors and sleep deprivation, research on, 106
  holistic care, xiv, 110–11
  hope-centric care, 195–97
  patients' fears, 125–26
  resilience training and, xix
  resiliency stories of, 139–41, 230–31
  role in lifestyle changes, 38–40, 96–98
  sense of purpose in, 230–33
  spirituality inventory and, 204–7
dopamine, 124, 156, 180
Dweck, Carol, 84

echocardiogram (ECG), 31–32
Edward (resiliency story), 164–65
Ekman, Paul, 120–21
Emily (resiliency story), 136
emotional intelligence, 13, 25
emotional pain, 178, 183
emotional regulation, 25, 93, 104, 136, 149, 156, 182
emotional self-care, 185–86
endocrine system, 19–20
The End of Trauma (Bonanno), 26
endorphins, 24, 90, 93, 95
epicardial cell regeneration, 181
epigenetics, 224
epinephrine. *see* adrenaline
Essential Principles of Resilience, 12–14
eustress. *see* good stress
excitement, effects on heart, 123–24
exercise and fitness. *see also* lifestyle choices; nutrition and diet
  aerobic exercise guidelines, 30, 32, 93–94
  grief effect on, 178

Index

in heart attack recovery standard of care, 90–93
in lessening anxiety and panic, 118–19
mental and physical benefits of, 6, 93–95
placebo effect and efficacy of, 80
resiliency story, 87–90
self-care and, 185
sense of purpose and, 223, 225
sleep and timing of, 107
exposure therapy, 118–19, 132, 136

faith and spirituality. *see also* hope
defining, 199
doctor-patient discussions and, 200–204
health outcomes and, 199–202
religious practices and mental health, 199–200, 202
in resilience-building in children, 10
self-care and, 186
spirituality inventory, 204–7
fatigue, as symptom, 32, 42, 88
fats (nutrient), 100, 102
fear, 117–38. *see also* anxiety
anxiety vs., 133–34
in Charney resilience principles, 13
chronic fear and effect on heart, 122–23
emotional and physiological components of, 119–21
heart attack recurrence fear, 117–19
moving forward in face of, 3, 126–29
resiliency stories, 124–26, 130–32
treatment and tools to manage, 134–38
FICA rubric, for spirituality inventory, 205–6
fight, flight, or freeze response, 19–20, 35, 56–57, 148–49, 156
flexible mindset, 63–85
in changing career path, 68–71
in denying limits after diagnosis, 73–77
nocebo effect and, 82–83
placebo effect and, 77–82

psychological flexibility and, 48–49, 73
resiliency stories, 2–3, 63–68, 71–72
in stress "perception" and effects of, 83–85
Francisco, Gerard, 113
Frankl, Viktor, and *Man's Search for Meaning*, 221
Friedman, Michael, 196–97
Fuster, Valentin, 128

Galatzer-Levy, Robert, 11–12
Garmezy, Norman, 8–9
Gary (resiliency story), 43–44
generosity, 172–73
George Washington Institute for Spirituality & Health, 205
Geronimus, Arline, 37–38
Gershman, Suzy, 113
ghrelin (hormone), 81–82
Gibran, Kahlil, 212
Giffords, Gabby, 112–14, 233
Global Epidemiology (journal), 194–95
glucose levels, 21, 89, 94, 100, 223
goal-setting, 13, 137
good stress, 23–24, 30, 33, 87, 118
Go Red for Women, 163
Grant, W. T., 154–55
Grant Study of Adult Development (1938), 154–55
grief
ambiguous grief, 60–61
finding purpose through, 225–26
intractable grief, 26
as love, 176–77
moving forward with loss, 58–60
processing feelings, 55–58
resilience strategies, 51–55
spousal death and health effects of, 177–80
Groban, Josh, "Granted," 236
gun violence, 112–14, 225–26, 230–31
Gupta, Sanjay, 218, 219
Gus (resiliency story), 168–70, 234

Index

habit formation, 108–15
Harold (resiliency story), 31–33
Harvard Study of Adult Development, 173
Harvard University, 154–55, 177, 202
Hawkley, Louise, 146–47
Hayes, Steven, 48–49, 73
Health Psychology (journal), 183
Healthy Cities (WHO), 184
heart
    electrical system of, xii, xiv, 18, 213
    fear response and effect on, 122–23
    oxytocin benefits to, 180–82
    structure and mechanics of, xii–xiii
heart attacks. *see also* cardiovascular disease
    cardiophobia and, 122
    causes of, 17–18
    fear of recurrence, 117–18
    grief and, 177, 179–80
    shifting standard of care for, 90–92
    widow-maker, 130
    in women, 16, 41–42
    heart-muscle injury, 101
heart rate, 21, 33, 149
heart surgery, xiii, 4–5, 43–44, 164–65
heart transplantation, 1–3, 5–6, 217
Heger, Astrid, 143, 144–45, 161, 197–98, 209
Hellerstein, Herman, 92
hippocampus, 25, 27–28, 29, 93, 149
hobbies, resilience and, 10, 185
holistic care, xiv–xv, 4–5, 110–11, 114–15, 196
Holt-Lunstad, Julianne, 170–71
homeostasis, 19, 20, 21–22, 24, 93, 122
Hone, Lucy, 51–55, 58–59, 61
hope. *see also* faith and spirituality
    assessments, 193–94
    defining, 192–93, 199
    health outcomes and, 3, 191–92, 194–95
    hope-centric care, 195–97
    resiliency stories, 197–98, 209
HOPE, for patient discussions, 200–201
hormone levels
    exercise and, 90, 93, 94
    nocebo effect and, 83
    nutrition and, 100, 102
    placebo effect and, 78
    stress and, 19–20, 21, 24–25
Horowitz, Carol, 231–32
hospice vs. palliative care, 66
HPA axis (hypothalamic-pituitary-adrenocortical axis), 19, 147, 148, 158
Huberman Lab (podcast), 82
hydration, 103, 185
hypertension. *see also* blood pressure
    chronic high blood pressure, 22
    chronic stress and, 33
    lifestyle changes for, 38–40
    stages of, 97
    weight and, 100
hypervigilance, 9, 21
hypothalamus, 19–20

immune system
    ambiguous loss and, 60
    exercise benefits to, 93, 94
    good stress and, 24
    grief effect on, 178
    loneliness effect on, 147, 148
    malnutrition and, 102
    placebo effect and, 78
    racial discrimination and, 16
    sense of purpose beneficial to, 224
    sleep and function of, 105
An Impossible Life (Wasden and Siddoway), 233
inequities, in healthcare system, 15–16
infant mortality rates, racial disparities and, 37
inflammation
    aerobic exercise in reducing, 93, 94
    excess weight and, 100
    inadequate sleep and, 105
    loneliness effects on, 147–49

Index

sense of purpose and, 224
stress and, 33
initiation phase, in habit formation, 109
insomnia, 149, 178
Institute for Disaster Mental Health at SUNY, 27
insulin resistance, 93, 100
Interfaculty Initiative on Health, Spirituality, and Religion (Harvard), 202
interpersonal neurobiology, 158–59
The Invisible String (book), 188–89
ischemia, 31–32

JAMA publications (Journal of the American Medical Association), 16, 152, 177
Jastreboff, Ania, 109–10
Jeff (resiliency story), 198
Jennifer (resiliency story), 197–98, 209
Johns Hopkins University, 101, 230
journaling, 178, 185
Journal of Advanced Nursing, 195
Journal of Health Psychology, 182–83
Journal of the American Heart Association, 16, 184
Joy in Medicine program, of AMA, 232
Julie (Narula friend), 144

Keck School of Medicine (University of Southern California), 71, 144
Kelly, Mark, 113
kindness, 159–60, 162, 180
Koenig, Harold, 202
Koh, Howard, 202
Kruse, Fabiane "Fabi" Hirsch, 113

Langer, Ellen, 80
Leahy, Robert, 134
learning phase, in habit formation, 109
Lenox Hill Hospital (New York), 204, 218–19
Levine, Alexandra, 191–92, 196–97

Levine, Samuel, and chair experiment, 91–92
Lewine, Howard, 179
life expectancy, 34–36
Life's Essential 8, 106
lifestyle choices. *see also* exercise and fitness; nutrition and diet; sleep
blood pressure and, 33, 38–40
cardiac rehab programs on, 184
challenges in making, 98–99
CVD, preventing and managing, 3, 17, 32–33
CVD diagnosis and, 42, 44–45
doctors' role in, 38–40, 96–98
habit formation and, 108–15
post-heart attack, 131
self-compassion and healthy habits, 182–83
sense of purpose and favorable lifestyle, 223, 225
Likert, Rensis, and Likert scale, 106
limbic system, 19, 104
Lisa and Bob (resiliency story), 174–75
loneliness and social isolation. *see also* building connections
mental health effects of, 149–51
mortality and, 147, 151, 170–71
physiological effects of, 147–49
spousal death and, 178
surgeon general on epidemic of, 151–52, 154–55
tools to counter, 155–65
in young adults, 152–54
"The Loneliness Epidemic Persists" (Cigna report), 152
Lopez, Shane, 194
Loprete, Denielle (resiliency story), 203–4
love, 167–89
defining, 167–68
effects on our brains and bodies, 171–79
grief and, 176–79. *see also* grief
heart health and, 179–82

Index

love (*cont.*)
  loving relationships and resilience, 4, 187–89
  resilience-love connection, 168–71
  resiliency stories, 174–76
  self-compassion and self-care as protective, 182–87
Lown, Bernard, 91–92

macronutrients and micronutrients, 102–3
malnutrition, 101–2
marriage, 173–80
Mary (resiliency story), 38–40
Maslow, Abraham, 7–8
Masten, Ann, 15
"Maternal Care and Mental Health" (Bowlby), 142
Mayo Clinic, 103
Mayo Clinic Proceedings (journal), 228
McGonigal, Kelly, 83–85, 94, 121–22
medical diagnosis
  acceptance in handling, 48–51
  cognitive reframing in managing, 137–38
  stress and trauma of receiving, xv, 40, 125
medical journalism, xii, xvi–xviii, 5–6, 12, 218–19
medical trauma, 4–5, 93, 115
medications, 42, 97, 109, 195
Medicine & Science in Sports & Exercise (journal), 94
meditation, 156, 185
Mediterranean diets, 103
memory, 25, 105, 149
mental health. *see also* anxiety; depression
  ambiguous loss and, 60
  cardiac rehabilitation focus on, 114–15
  CVD risk and, 18–19, 111
  exercise role in, 6, 93
  loneliness effects on, 147, 149–51
  marital satisfaction and, 173
  religious/spiritual practices and, 199–200, 202
  resiliency story, 233–34
  screen time increase and, 153–54
  self-care and, 183–86
mentalistic theory, 79
Merlis, Andy (resiliency story), 87–90
mesolimbic reward system, 173
metabolic systems and function, 22, 24, 81–82, 93–94, 100–101, 104–5, 110
Michigan State University, 181–82
"the milkshake" experiment, 81–82
Miller, BJ (resiliency story), 63–68, 71, 129, 209, 233
mind-body-spirit connection, 4–7, 204–7
Mindful Awareness Research Center (UCLA), 158
mindfulness practices, 45, 49, 134, 156, 178, 185
ministrokes, 71–72
minorities, healthcare inequities and, 15–16
Miriam (resiliency story), 55–60, 121
"The Moment I Knew Medicine Was My Calling" (AMA series), 232–33
Moms Demand Action, 225
mood, effects on, 25, 34, 90, 94–95, 159, 160, 173, 181
Mood and Anxiety Research Program (National Institute of Mental Health), 12
mortality
  CVD as leading cause of death, xiii, 17
  facing fear of, 128–29
  factors in reducing risk of, 194, 223, 224
  loneliness and, 147, 151, 170–71
  widowhood effect and, 177
Mount Sinai Hospital (New York)
  Center for Stress, Resilience and Personal Growth, 14–15, 137, 228
  Fuster Heart Hospital of, 128
  Icahn School of Medicine, 13–14, 164, 231
  9/11 mental health program, 28
"moving the goalposts," 54

Index

multiple sclerosis, 73–77
Murthy, Vivek, 151–52, 160, 229, 232
myocardial infarction (MI). *see* heart attacks
myokines, 94–95

Narula, Tara. *see also* doctors and healthcare providers
   connection with mentor, 161–63
   exercise preferences of, 95
   father's medical career and resilience story, xiv, 213–17
   finding purpose as a doctor, xiv–xv, 212–19
   flexible mindset in career path of, 68–71
   heart transplant patient and, 1–3, 5–6, 217
   medical journalism and, xii, xvi–xviii, 5–6, 12, 218–19
   mother's lesson on imprint of small interactions, 208–9
   noninvasive cardiology and holistic care of patients, xii, xiv–xv
   personal love-resilience connection, 167–68
   on power of resilience, 235–36
   on value of connection in medical field, 143–46
   vision loss and acceptance, 45–48
National Center for Health Statistics, 36
National Center for PTSD, 25, 29
National Institute on Aging, 151
National Institutes of Health (NIH), 67
National Poll on Healthy Aging, in *JAMA*, 152
NBC Nightly News, 218
neurocardiology, 123
neuroendocrine system, 19–20
neurogenesis, slowing of, 25
neuroplasticity, 23, 93, 149, 156, 179
neurotransmitters, 19, 78, 79, 149, 156
9/11 attacks and responders, 12, 27, 28
nocebo effect, 82–83
norepinephrine, 124, 148

NRA (National Rifle Association), 231
nutrition and diet
   body mass index, 99–101
   grief effect on, 178
   healthy eating habits, 101–4
   placebo effect and "milkshake" experiment, 81–82
   self-care and, 185
   stress effects on, 25
   weight control, 100–102

obesity, 100–101, 109–10, 147
Office of Disease Prevention and Health Promotion (ODPHP), 30, 32
optimism, 6, 11, 13, 192. *see also* hope
Otto, Michael, 118
Our Epidemic of Loneliness and Isolation (surgeon general report), 152, 154
overeating, as stress response, 110
The Oxford Handbook of Positive Psychology, 194
oxytocin, 156, 158, 180–82

Paige (resiliency story), 50–51
palliative care, 66–67
Palmer, Julie, 16
panic attacks, 48–49, 56–58, 118–19
parent-child bond, 188–89
pathways, in theory of hope, 193
Pavlovian theory, 79
perceived social isolation, 147
personality, resilience and, 9
Peter Bent Brigham Hospital (Boston), 91
physical touch, 157–58, 180–81
Physician Well-Being Program, of AMA, 232
pituitary gland, 19–20
placebo effect, 199
"Plan of the Master Weaver" (poem), 208–9
plaque buildup. *see* atherosclerosis
Pollan, Michael, 104
positive psychology, 7–8

Index

Posttraumatic Growth Inventory (PTGI), 11
potentially traumatic events (PTEs), 11
poverty, chronic stress and, 36–37
prefrontal cortex, 25, 29, 93, 104, 149
pre-purposes, 220
primates, stress adaptability in, 21
Principles of Medical Ethics (of AMA), 172
processed foods, xiv, 98, 103–4, 105
Proenza, Mrs. (teacher), 218
proto-purposes, 220
psychological first aid, 27–29
psychological flexibility
   TEDx Talk on, 48–49
   three pillars of, 73
"Psychological Health, Well-Being, and the Mind-Heart-Body-Connection," 111
Psychological Science (journal), 80
psychological stress, 21–22
Psychology, Health & Medicine (journal), 108–9
Psychosomatic Medicine (journal), 223–24
PTEs (potentially traumatic events), 11
PTGI (Posttraumatic Growth Inventory), 11
PTSD (post-traumatic stress disorder), 14–15, 25–30, 119
Puchalski, Christina, 205
purpose, 211–34
   burnout in healthcare workers and, 227–30, 232
   emergence of, 219–20, 225–27
   finding our "why," 3, 211–12
   health benefits, 223–25
   in keeping doctors motivated, 230–33
   Narula's career path and father's role in, 212–19. *see also* Narula, Tara
   resiliency story, 233–34
   scales and assessments in measuring, 220–23
   self-care and, 186, 225
Purpose in Life test, 221

racial discrimination, 16, 37
radical acceptance, 171–72, 234
Raz, Guy, on NPR, 122
recognizing strengths, as resilience principle, 13
Reeve, Christopher and Dana, 175–76
regenerative medicine, 182
relaxation techniques, 107, 134, 178
religion. *see* faith and spirituality
reproductive system, 20, 148
resilience, defined, xvi–xvii
resilience paradox, 27
resilience psychology, history of, 7–16
Resilience Response
   acceptance and, 41–61. *see also* acceptance
   building connections with others, 139–65. *see also* building connections
   Essential Principles of Resilience, 12–14
   facing fear, 117–38. *see also* fear
   flexible thinking and, 63–85. *see also* flexible mindset
   hope and faith in, 191–209. *see also* faith and spirituality; hope
   love and, 167–89
   mind, body and spirit in building resilience, 4–7
   origins of, xvii–xviii, 1–16
   physical health and, 87–115. *See also* exercise and fitness; lifestyle choices; nutrition and diet; sleep
   psychology of resilience, xvi, 7–16
   pushing forward with resilience, 235–36
   sense of purpose in, 211–34. *see also* purpose
   stress and, 8–9, 17–40. *see also* stress
Resilient Grieving (Hone), 55
rest-and-digest mode, 156
reward system (brain), 110, 124, 156, 172–73
Riegel, Barbara, 184
role models and mentors, 10, 13
Romanian adoptees, study on resilience in, 9

Index

runner's high, 94–95, 180
Rutter, Michael, 9
Ryff, Carol D., and Ryff Inventory, 222

Sakran, Joseph, 230–31
Salk, Jonas, 196
Samuels, Martin, 123
Sapolsky, Robert, 20–22
schizophrenia, 8
Scioli, Anthony, 199
self-care, 183–87
self-compassion, 182–83
Self-Compassion Scale, 183
"Sense of Purpose Moderates the Associations Between Daily Stressors and Daily Well-Being," 224
Sense of Purpose Scale, 221–22
September 11, 2001. *see* 9/11 attacks and responders
Serenity Prayer, 47, 48
The Shawshank Redemption, on hope, 192
Shear, Katherine, 176–77
shortness of breath, 18, 31, 32, 42, 56
shoulder, neck, or jaw pain, 42
Shulman, Lisa M., 177–79
sick sinus syndrome, 203
Siegel, Dan, 158
Singh, Dr., 204
Sinha, Michael S., 232–33
sleep
  ambiguous loss and, 60
  brain health and, 104–5
  chronic stress and, 34
  grief effects on, 178
  loneliness effect on, 147, 149
  quality-sleep tips, 107–8
  self-care and, 185
  sleep deprivation effects, 105–6
  stress effects on, 25
Smith, Ruth, 9–10
Smits, Jasper, 118
smoking, 39–40, 114, 223
Snyder, C. R., 193–94

social anxiety, 119, 147
social inequity, stress of, 36–38
social interactions. *see* building connections
social isolation. *see* loneliness and social isolation
Society of General Internal Medicine, 231–32
Song, Kristin, Ethan's Law and, 225–26
Southwick, Steven, 10
spirituality inventory, 204–7. *see also* faith and spirituality
spousal death, effects of, 177–80
stability phase, in habit formation, 109
Stanford, Fatima Cody, 233
Stanford University, 68–70, 79, 228
stents, 32, 88, 89, 130, 204
stress, 17–40
  brain health and, 22–30
  CVD prevention and, 17–18
  exercise in mitigating effects of, 93–96
  fear vs., 121
  flexible mindset and effects of, 83–85
  grief-induced, 177–78
  health effects of, 34–38
  heart and, 30–34
  loneliness as stressor, 147–51
  negatives and positives of, 18–20
  resiliency story, 38–40
  self-compassion as protective, 182–83
  sense of purpose in regulation of, 224
  trauma and effects on brain, 25–29
  types of, 20–22. *see also* acute stress; chronic stress
stress adaptation, 8–9
stress cardiomyopathy (broken heart syndrome), xiii, 179–80
Stress First Aid program (Northwell hospital system), 28–29
stress-response system, 11, 19–24, 147–48
strokes, 17–18, 33, 71–72, 147, 149, 177. *see also* cardiovascular disease
substance use, 49, 223, 225
Sun Juice, 69–71

Index

Super/Man: The Christopher Reeve Story (documentary), 175–76
support network, resilience and, 9, 13
sympathetic nervous system, 148–49
systolic blood pressure, 97, 184

takotsubo cardiomyopathy (broken heart syndrome), xiii, 179–80
Tedeschi, Richard, 10–11, 12
teens and adolescents, 6, 49–50, 152–53, 220
This Is Our Lane (online community), 231
Thought Record (CBT exercise), 134–35
"Three Secrets of Resilient People" (2019 TED Talk), 51–52
Thurston, Rebecca C., 183
TIAs (transient ischemic attacks), 71–72
Tippett, Krista, 65
Together: The Healing Power of Human Connection in a Sometimes Lonely World (Murthy), 160
touch, 157–58, 180–81
transient stress, 26
trauma
  in building resilience, 10–12
  COVID pandemic and, 14
  finding purpose in, 225–26
  goal-setting in overcoming, 13
  of heart attack/surgery, 131
  medical diagnosis as, xv, 125
  medical trauma, 4–5, 93, 115
  PTSD, 14–15, 25–30, 119
  stress and effects on brain, 25–29
triglyceride levels, 100
troponin, 101

University of Michigan, 37
University of Wisconsin-Madison, 84
US Department of Health, 229
US surgeon general advisories, 151–52, 229, 232

VanderWeele, Tyler, 202
ventricular fibrillation, 122–23

Vieira, Meredith, 74, 75
Violence Intervention Program (VIP), 145
Viscott, David, 234
La vita è bella (Roberto Benigni film), 235
volunteering, 163, 180, 186

Waldinger, Robert, 155, 159
Walters, Barbara, 76
Wasden, Sonja (resiliency story), 233–34
Weathering: The Extraordinary Stress of Ordinary Life in an Unjust Society (Geronimus), 37–38
weathering hypothesis, 37–38
weight management, 94, 100–102
Weiner, Bill, 178
Werner, Emmy, 9–10
White, Paul Dudley, 92
Why Zebras Don't Get Ulcers (Sapolsky), 20–21
widowhood effect, 177
widow-maker (heart attack), 130
Williams, Daniel Hale, xiii
Williams, Michelle, 36
Williams, Robin, 146
Winshall, James "Jamie," 162–63
women
  broken heart syndrome in, 179–80
  CVD symptoms in, 41–42
  Go Red for Women initiative, 163
  healthcare inequities and, 15–16
  value of connection among, 143–46
Women's Biobehavioral Health Program (University of Pittsburgh), 183
World Health Organization (WHO), 27, 66, 183–84, 227
World Trade Center Health Program, 28

Yale Center for Clinical and Translational Research, 81
Yale Obesity Research Center, 109

About the Author

Dr. Tara Narula is a board-certified cardiologist at Lenox Hill Hospital in Manhattan, an associate professor of cardiovascular medicine at the Zucker School of Medicine, Hofstra/Northwell, the associate director of the Women's Heart Program at Lenox Hill Hospital, and director of communications for the Katz Institute of Women's Health. She is also a nationally recognized medical journalist. She is the current chief medical correspondent for ABC News and a former NBC News medical contributor, CNN medical correspondent, and CBS News senior medical correspondent. She has been a past contributor as well to *O, The Oprah Magazine*. She joined Lenox Hill Heart & Vascular Institute of New York in 2010 and provides outpatient consultative care. After graduating from Stanford University with degrees in economics and biology, she was founder and CEO of her own small business, Sun Juice Inc. Subsequently she obtained her medical degree at the University of Southern California Keck School of Medicine, where she graduated with Alpha Omega Alpha Society honors. Dr. Narula completed her residency in internal medicine at Harvard University/Brigham and Women's Hospital and her fellowship

About the Author

training in cardiology at New York Presbyterian-Weill Cornell Medical Center. Dr. Narula is currently a fellow of the American College of Cardiology (FACC). She serves as a national spokesperson for the American Heart Association and the AHA's Go Red for Women Initiative. She is codirector of a mentoring program for women in medicine called Face of Cardiology, which serves to help guide women pursuing possible careers in cardiology. She is a recipient of a 2022 Emmy Award for Outstanding Live News Program CBS Mornings, the 2019 WomenHeart Nanette Wenger Award for Media, and the Super Doctors Award for NYC 2014–2025. Her interests include women's health, prevention, mental health, and resilience.